"A Must"

"*Optimal Muscle Recovery* is a must for coaches and athletes. It contains a lot of important information on how to maximize your training and excel in your sport. The book makes you understand how important recovery is for your athletic success. I wish this kind of knowledge was available when I was competing."

Grete Waitz
Nine-time Winner of the New York City Marathon

"Highly Recommended"

"A simple but dramatic approach to improved training, fitness, and recovery that anyone can follow on a daily basis. Highly recommended."

Bob Anderson
Author of *Stretching*

"Important"

"Recovery is the most important issue that my athletes face while training hard. This book contains key concepts that I now use to help them speed their recovery and optimize their training."

Chris Carmichael
1996 Olympic Cycling Team Head Coach

"Invaluable"

"Ed Burke unveils the latest clinical yet practical nutritional truths about muscle recovery. The book will be an invaluable training and racing tool for all athletes and coaches who have questioned the validity of optimum dietary supplementation to enhance performance. *Optimal Muscle Recovery* is a fantastic addition to my health library."

Dave Scott
Six-time Winner of the Ironman Triathlon

"Read This Book"

"Recovery, often neglected by both the recreational and elite athlete, is one of the keys to continual improvement in sport. In *Optimal Muscle Recovery*, Ed Burke shows the reader how and why to utilize the R^4 System of recovery for improved athletic success. What could be easier? If you want to train and compete at a higher level, read this book and put it to use!"

Harvey Newton
CSCS Executive Director,
National Strength & Conditioning Association Coach
USA Weightlifting Team, 1984 Olympic Games

"World-Class"

"It's no longer enough to train hard—recovery is emerging as the real key to athletic improvement. Ed Burke's new book shows you how to take maximum advantage of those grueling workouts with world-class recovery techniques."

Fred Matheny
Fitness Editor for *Bicycling Magazine*

"Very Understandable"

"Dr. Ed Burke has made a major contribution to the science of recovery. He outlines in a very understandable fashion the current body of scientific knowledge with regard to renewing muscle fibers. His four simple principles, incorporated into the R^4 System, explain the process. It's not magic—it's scientifically based and it makes sense."

Frank Shorter
Olympic Marathon Gold and Silver Medalist

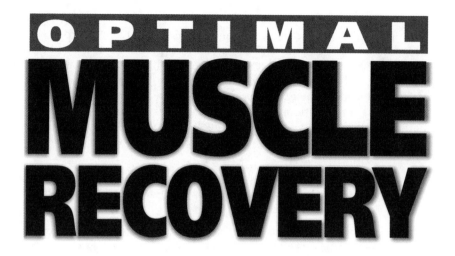

OPTIMAL MUSCLE RECOVERY

Edmund R. Burke, PhD

AVERY PUBLISHING GROUP

Garden City Park • New York

The information and advice contained in this book are based upon the research and the personal and professional experiences of the author. They are not intended as a substitute for consulting with a health care professional. The publisher and author are not responsible for any adverse effects or consequences resulting from the use of any of the suggestions, preparations, or procedures discussed in this book. All matters pertaining to your physical health should be supervised by a health care professional. It is a sign of wisdom, not cowardice, to seek a second or third opinion.

The R^{4TM} System is a registered trademark of Edmund R. Burke, PhD.

Cover designer: Eric Macaluso
In-house editor: Peggy Hahn
Typesetter: Gary A. Rosenberg
Illustrator (Chapter 15): John Wincek
Printer: Paragon Press, Honesdale, PA

Avery Publishing Group
120 Old Broadway
Garden City Park, NY 11040
1-800-548-5757
www.averypublishing.com

Cataloging-in-Publication Data

Burke, Ed, 1949-
    Optimal muscle recovery / Edmund R. Burke;
Foreword by Frank Shorter.
    p. cm.
    Includes bibliographical references and index.
    ISBN: 0-89529-884-8

    1. Sports medicine. 2. Exercise—Physiological
aspects. 3. Muscles—Motility. I. Title.

RC1236.M8B87 1999   617.1'027
                                       QBI99-305

Printed in the United States of America

10 9 8 7 6 5 4 3 2 1

CONTENTS

Part III: Going the Extra Mile

ACKNOWLEDGMENTS

I am grateful to the many dedicated people whose hard work and support made this project possible. First, thanks to Robert Portman, Ph.D., for hosting and supporting the symposium that led to the creation of this book. It was obvious after listening to the guest speakers that there was a better nutritional regimen to help athletes improve athletic performance.

I would like to thank Drs. John Ivy and Robert Kaman, as well as Dr. Portman, for their careful critiquing and editing of the book. Thanks also to Drs. John Seifert and Peter Raven, and to all the students in their laboratories, who worked on the research presented in this book.

My heartfelt thanks to Tracy Scarpa for her ability to pull together all the edits of the manuscript. I would also like to thank the good people at Avery Publishing, and in particular my editor, Peggy Hahn. Without her steady and professional editorial hand to guide and shape the final presentation of the manuscript, it would never have come to fruition.

My deepest gratitude goes out to all the athletes I have worked with over the last twenty years, who have given me the insight to look beyond "traditional" nutritional information and research to find the truth behind sports nutrition. I am also indebted to the many scientists, nutritionists, and medical professionals who are expanding the frontiers of our knowledge of nutrition, antioxidants, herbs, and carbohydrate and protein supplementation. We are very fortunate to have these dedicated men and women waging the war against complacency in nutrition research and education.

Above all, I am thankful to have a wonderful wife, Kathleen, who understands the long hours it takes to write books of this nature. She has always been there to support my efforts.

There are many others, too numerous to name, who have guided, advised, and supported me as I put this book together. I owe them all a debt of gratitude for helping me to produce a guide that will be helpful to you, my reader, and to the athletes you work with on the field or in the gym.

FOREWORD

We all want to get the most out of our training programs. Some of us exercise for fitness, others train for competition, but all of us push our bodies to the limit—sometimes daily—in order to maximize our workouts. As dedicated athletes, we may put in several hours at a time of strenuous exercise to improve beyond base conditioning, and to develop strength and endurance. But intense, exhaustive exercise is only one aspect of an effective training program.

Successful athletes and their coaches and trainers know that it's impossible to train extremely hard on consecutive days for any extended period of time. This is especially true for endurance runners. Our bodies need approximately twenty-four to thirty-six hours to recover from strenuous training. These days, a "hard-easy" schedule, which incorporates easy days of less intense training, is an accepted part of every smart endurance athlete's routine. It's as simple as listening to your body. You know when you have maximized your workout or raced to your limit because your body will not allow you to continue, and you won't be able to go at the same level the next day—no matter how hard you try.

Optimal Muscle Recovery is a breakthrough contribution to the science of recovery from exercise. For years now we have been aware of the importance of replacement drinks to restore the body's balance of fluids and salts, such as sodium, potassium, and magnesium. Dr. Edmund Burke has taken the idea of restoring balance to a new level. In this book, he teaches us that returning to a state of balance also involves replenishing energy stores and rebuilding damaged muscle fibers. With his revolutionary R^4 System, Dr. Burke has interpreted the current body of scientific knowledge into four remarkably simple principles that will help you maximize your recovery from exercise. The secret to complete recovery lies in carefully balanced nutrition and nutritional supplementation that will enable you to reduce muscle damage, restore energy, and regain your strength after exercise. When you help your body make a full recovery, you'll find that it's easier to exercise at peak capacity in your next training session.

Reaching your performance goals takes time and a great deal of patience. You can't "magically" achieve the standards that you set for yourself without hard work and perseverance. But *Optimal Muscle Recovery* presents real-world, practical guidelines that can help you get started on the road to peak performance.

Frank Shorter

INTRODUCTION

I started to study exercise physiology and sports nutrition in the 1970s, with the conviction that proper nutrition, in addition to a good training program, is crucial for optimal performance. In the years since then, I have had the good fortune to work with a number of the world's leading sports scientists, and to collaborate with them on studies that have defined a new vision of sports nutrition.

Much of the research conducted in the last two decades has focused on gaining a greater understanding of the body's physiological responses to dehydration, and the impact of carbohydrate supplementation—prior to and during exercise—on performance. Studies on carbohydrate, in particular, have highlighted the effects of pre-exercise energy stores on endurance performance, which has resulted in a popular practice known as carbohydrate loading. Sports scientists and nutritionists have also investigated the roles of other basic nutrients, such as protein and fat, in fueling exercise. The culmination of this research has been the establishment of guidelines for an effective athletic diet.

Only in the last few years, however, have we begun to

investigate the role of nutrition in helping muscles *recover* from exercise lasting more than sixty minutes, generally referred to as long-term exercise. Because most of your muscles' adaptations for increased strength and endurance occur in the interval between exercise sessions, your ability to perform at a high level day after day is limited by the extent of muscle recovery and repair after strenuous training. Therefore, it's no longer enough to train long and hard—you have to train smart.

"Take rest and recovery nutrition as seriously as you take your training. For the most part, strength and endurance capacity are developed not during the training session, but instead during the rest phase, when the muscle tissue grows stronger," says Jay T. Kearney, Ph.D., Exercise Physiologist at the Olympic Training Center in Colorado Springs, Colorado. It has become quite clear that providing the right nutrients in the right proportions before, during, and after exercise ensures your muscles' health and increases endurance capacity and strength, all of which lead to improved performance. Not only should you replenish your body's depleted energy stores, but you also have to take steps to minimize and repair damaged muscle tissue. Sports nutrition research now provides us with guidance to achieve this goal.

In 1997, I participated in a symposium in Colorado Springs, attended by top exercise physiologists. The objective of the symposium was to review the most recent studies on enhancing recovery both during and after exercise. It was during this symposium that the R^4 System for Peak Performance was developed, with the basic goal to help athletes achieve full muscle potential through a comprehensive recovery program.

Based on the latest research on muscle performance and recovery, the R^4 System is an important milestone in our understanding of exercise physiology. It highlights the importance of energy replacement during and after exercise to extend performance, and focuses on minimizing and repairing exercise-induced muscle damage in order to maintain muscle strength. The R^4 System establishes four simple, practical principles that all endurance athletes can incorporate into their daily training. If you want to optimize recovery and achieve full muscle potential, you should:

- **Restore** fluids and important minerals to recover from dehydration,

- **Replenish** glycogen, a primary fuel source for energy,

- **Reduce** muscle and immune-system damage resulting from the physical stress of exercise, and

- **Rebuild** muscle protein, which is important for the maintenance of muscle structure and function.

Optimal Muscle Recovery will dramatically change the way you train and prepare for competition. Part I lays the groundwork in clear, understandable terms by reviewing basic muscle structure and function. You'll learn about the essential nutrients that your body uses for energy, and the three possible ways in which your muscles "burn" these nutrients for fuel. This is followed by a comprehensive look at the causes of muscle fatigue and exercise-induced muscle damage. Finally, Part I establishes the foundation for the R^4 System by explaining the processes involved in recovery from exercise.

Part II is the heart of the book because it details each of the four components of the R^4 System. You'll discover how to maximize recovery by making some surprisingly simple changes in your exercise-nutrition program. And each chapter provides you with guidelines that will enable you to tailor these revolutionary nutritional principles to suit your body's needs. This part of the book also explains how exercise physiologists have made science practical by developing a new sports nutrition product based upon the latest research on recovery.

The last part of *Optimal Muscle Recovery* takes you beyond the R^4 System by outlining other measures that will help you enhance performance and maintain overall health. Part III provides an overview of general nutrition for maximal performance in your everyday activities, even when you're not exercising. Following this is a discussion of cutting-edge nutritional supplements that athletes who are "in the know" are using to optimize recovery, from well-known creatine and caffeine to lesser known phosphatidylserine and ribose. This final part also shows you how to stockpile your energy stores through carbohydrate loading prior to intense exercise or competition—without suffering from common side effects such as heaviness in the limbs. Last but not least, you'll find important information on nonnutritional approaches to recovery, from pre- and post-competition massage to sessions in the sauna or hot tub to stretching techniques.

The goal of this book is to help you better understand how exercise affects your muscles, and how taking measures to ensure proper recovery can counteract some of the consequences of strenuous training or competition. You will learn how to extend performance, maintain muscle strength, and develop your muscles day by day. By adopting the R^4 System for Peak Performance, you'll feel healthier and perform at a higher level than you ever thought possible. Let *Optimal Muscle Recovery* show you how.

PART I

MUSCLE PERFORMANCE BASICS

Whether you're a professional athlete or a "week-end warrior," you probably know what it's like to run out of steam during strenuous exercise. Or maybe, the day after intense training, you are reminded by your sore, stiff muscles that you had better take it easy next time. Most athletes accept these consequences of exercise as inevitable. Many, in fact, take these signs to mean that they are not training hard enough, and concentrate on increasing the difficulty or duration of their workouts. The problem with this approach, however, is that it does not address the underlying causes of muscle fatigue and soreness. Learning how to minimize these discomforts is as simple as understanding how your muscles work, and how exercise affects their structure and function.

Part I reviews the mechanics and chemistry behind muscle contraction, from the physical structure of human skeletal muscle, to the way your body uses carbohydrate, fat, and protein to synthesize energy for all of its activities. It then builds upon this information to explain how exercise affects your muscles on the physical and biochemical levels, causing fatigue and muscle damage. And, most important, this first part explains the three critical phases of recovery, during which time your body returns to a state of balance, replenishes depleted energy stores, and repairs damaged muscle tissue.

1.

HOW MUSCLES WORK

Many people are of the opinion that well-developed muscles are the most visible testament to physical fitness. Firm, toned muscles are aesthetically pleasing, and millions of us dedicate hours each day to exercise in an effort to appear "muscular." However, we have to look beyond size—the most obvious aspect of muscles—to understand muscular fitness. The most important aspect of our muscle system is function.

Muscles are highly specialized tissues that can contract to produce body movement. They enable us to carry out the innumerable functions that are essential to daily life. Yet, most people don't know about the underlying physiology of the human muscle system. This is because our actions are generated so quickly that we're not aware of the complicated processes behind them.

To understand how muscle recovery is key to peak muscle performance during exercise, you should have some background knowledge about how your muscles work. This chapter reviews basic muscle structure and function.

THE THREE TYPES OF MUSCLE TISSUE

Muscle tissue makes up a large part of the human body—
40 to 45 percent of a man's body by weight and 30 to 35
percent of a woman's body by weight. Of course, percentage of muscle weight is considerably higher in those athletes who train regularly and intensely, such as champion
bodybuilders. In total, your body contains some 650 muscles. About 620 of these muscles are called *skeletal muscles*
because they are fastened to the bones of your skeleton by
strong connective tissues known as tendons. The main
function of the skeletal muscle system is the voluntary
movement of the body. These muscles are classified as voluntary muscles because you can contract them at will.

The remaining muscles are composed of cardiac muscle
and smooth muscle. *Cardiac muscle,* or heart muscle, is
responsible for pumping blood through the body. *Smooth
muscle* is found in the walls of organs such as the stomach,
intestines, and urinary bladder, and in blood vessels.
Among its many other functions, smooth muscle helps
substances move through the intestinal tract, and also
changes the diameter of blood vessels. Because you cannot
control the contractions of your smooth muscles at will,
they are known as involuntary muscles.

THE STRUCTURE AND FUNCTION OF
SKELETAL MUSCLE

Skeletal muscle tissue is composed of bundles of long
fibers. Each fiber is actually a muscle cell, which is sur-
rounded by a thin membrane. Muscle cells are responsible
for producing the enormous amounts of energy that your
muscles require for contraction.

Figure 1.1 provides a closer look at the individual muscle fiber. As you can see, the cell consists of smaller units
called *myofibrils,* which are the structures directly involved

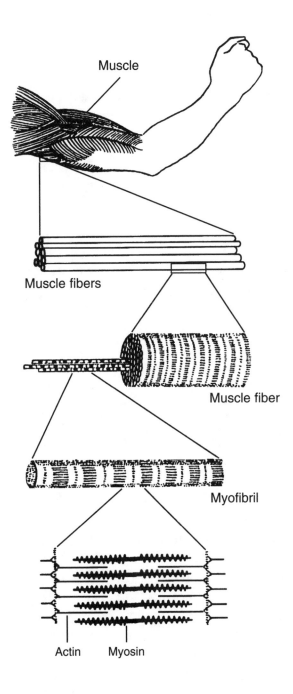

Muscle

Muscle fibers

Muscle fiber

Myofibril

Actin   Myosin

Figure 1.1. The structure of skeletal muscles

in contraction. Myofibrils can be divided further into thin and thick filaments, which are the proteins *actin* and *myosin*. The arrangement of these filaments is what gives your skeletal muscle tissue its striped, or *striated*, appearance. Muscular contraction is produced when the thin actin filaments slide across the thick myosin filaments, causing the muscle fiber to shorten.

Even the simplest muscle movement is produced by a complex series of operations. First, the order to contract is transmitted from your brain by your nerve cells to the appropriate muscle fiber. Then, the stimulus passes along the muscle fiber, causing the muscle to contract. This intricate series of actions takes only one one-thousandth of a second, making the response to the initial impulse seem almost instantaneous.

Fast- and Slow-Twitch Muscle Fibers

Although all skeletal muscles share the same properties, all skeletal muscle tissue is not the same. There are two general types of muscle fibers—fast-twitch and slow-twitch—and each has different structural and functional properties. *Fast-twitch* muscle fibers contract more quickly than slow-twitch fibers, but fatigue easily. *Slow-twitch* fibers, on the other hand, do not tire as easily, and are therefore used for high-endurance activities. Everybody has both types of fibers in their muscles, but the relative amount that a person has of each can vary widely. Some athletes, in fact, can have as much as 80 percent of one particular fiber type.

Fast-twitch fibers contract rapidly, and function well anaerobically, without a steady supply of oxygen. (Anaerobic metabolism will be discussed in greater detail in Chapter 2.) These are responsible for strength and speed in high-intensity, low-endurance activities that demand quick bursts of energy, such as sprinting, jumping, and shot-putting. They are also used for situations where stop-and-go movements are required, such as in basketball and volleyball. However, fast-twitch fibers fatigue quickly due to the buildup of *lactic acid,* a byproduct of anaerobic metabolism. Not surprisingly, athletes who excel in short-duration sports requiring a high-energy output seem to have a relatively large proportion of fast- to slow-twitch fibers.

Slow-twitch fibers use oxygen to produce a steady supply of energy for prolonged activity. These fibers function more slowly and are well suited to less intensive aerobic activities because they do not fatigue easily. (Aerobic metabolism will be discussed in greater detail in Chapter 2.) Slow-twitch fibers have large numbers of small blood vessels called *capillaries* to bring in oxygen and nutrients and to carry off waste products such as carbon dioxide. Therefore, they are advantageous for long-term training or competition. Athletes who excel at endurance sports have a higher proportion of slow-twitch fibers.

The proportion of fast- to slow-twitch muscle fibers in your muscles is determined by genetics, and is therefore fixed at birth. This means that the fiber ratio cannot be altered significantly by training. Elite athletes generally possess a greater quantity of one type of fiber. For instance, a marathon runner would possess more slow-twitch fibers than a 100-meter sprinter, while the sprinter would have a greater percentage of fast-twitch fibers. All muscle fibers, however, can respond to athletic training by improving their ability to perform.

HOW OPPOSING FORCES WORK TOGETHER

Muscles can forcefully contract, but they cannot forcefully expand. This means that when a muscle pulls a bone in one direction, it is unable to pull the bone back to its original position. For this reason, skeletal muscles function in opposing, or *antagonistic,* pairs.

Figure 1.2 illustrates how two muscles work against

each other to produce movements of the human arm. As shown below, the contraction of your biceps muscle, which is considered to be the *agonist,* allows you to raise your forearm in order to lift a weight. The shortening of the biceps muscle is known as *concentric contraction.* At the same time, the triceps muscle, known as the *antagonist,* extends.

In order to lower your arm, your triceps muscle (now the agonist) must contract. This contraction allows for the relaxation and extension of the biceps muscle (now the antagonist) to return your arm to its original position. In this case, the lengthening of the biceps muscle is called *eccentric contraction.*

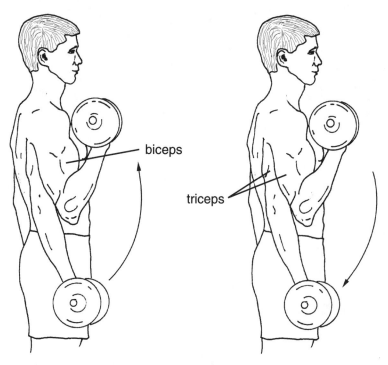

Figure 1.2. The figure on the left shows the concentric contraction of the biceps muscle, in which the biceps is the agonist, while the triceps muscle is the antagonist. The figure on the right shows the eccentric contraction of the biceps muscle, in which the triceps muscle is the agonist, and the biceps is the antagonist.

CONCLUSION

The architecture of your skeletal muscle system is extremely intricate. As you continue to read this book, try to notice some of the simple actions that your skeletal muscles perform—actions that you would normally take for granted, such as opening the book and turning its pages. Each and every movement of your body occurs through a series of precise operations, which begins with the command to contract from your brain, and results in the contraction of a muscle or group of muscles.

Now we can move on to examine what enables muscles to contract. The next chapter focuses on how your body produces the energy it needs for movement.

2.

The Energy Currency of Muscles

Muscle cells require extraordinary amounts of energy to contract—especially during exercise. To produce the energy your body needs, nature has designed an extremely sophisticated metabolic system. Energy is released when your muscle cells break down carbohydrate, fat, and protein. Your body uses these nutrients in specific proportions during exercise, depending on the length and intensity of your activity.

In this chapter, we will discuss the basic nutrients that provide you with necessary energy for training or competition. We will focus on the three energy pathways by which your body "burns" these fuels to release energy for muscle contraction.

MACRONUTRIENTS

Macronutrients are nutrients that your body requires daily in large amounts in order to function properly. These nutrients, including carbohydrate, fat, and protein, supply your body with energy, and serve as the building blocks for growth and repair.

The fourth and most important macronutrient, water, contains no calories, and does not provide energy in and of itself. However, it is a vital component in every function of the body, including all digestive, absorption, circulatory, and excretory functions. The role of this essential macronutrient will be discussed in greater detail in Chapter 3.

Carbohydrate

Carbohydrate is your body's most readily available source of nutrient energy. Through digestion and metabolism, carbohydrate is converted into *glucose* to be used as an immediate source of fuel. Glucose that is not used directly to provide energy is transported by the blood to your liver and muscle tissues, where it is converted into *glycogen* for storage. The hormone insulin, which is released from the pancreas, facilitates the transport of glucose from the blood to the sites of glycogen storage. However, the capacity of your liver and muscle tissues to store glycogen is limited. If you consume more carbohydrate than your body can use at that time, then some carbohydrate will be stored as fat in your adipose (fat) tissues.

During exercise, the stored glycogen in your muscle cells is broken down into glucose to manufacture *adenosine triphosphate* (ATP), which is the source of energy for all living cells. Through proper training, athletes can "teach" their muscles to store greater amounts of glycogen, and to conserve that glycogen so they will have increased energy reserves during exercise or competition. This philosophy of training is the basis for the practice of carbohydrate loading, which will be discussed later, in Chapter 14.

The intensity and duration of your activity determines how much glycogen your body uses during training or competition. For example, intense activities that demand a high output of energy in a short time frame, such as sprinting, quickly deplete your body's glycogen stores. Jogging, a less intense form of steady exercise, is more conservative. Glycogen is still used, but your reserves do not run out as quickly. Keep in mind, however, that the supply will eventually be exhausted.

Fat

Fat is your body's most concentrated source of food energy. Unlike the glycogen stored in your liver and muscle tissues, fat stores can fuel hours of exercise without running out. However, because the majority of fat is stored in the adipose tissue of your body, it is not as readily available for energy production as is carbohydrate. In order to be utilized for energy, fat molecules must first be broken down into *fatty acids*. Then, in this form, they are transported to your working muscles by the blood.

The duration of exercise directly influences how your body uses fat for energy. Fat can only be broken down for energy during low- to moderate-intensity, longer-duration aerobic exercise. Therefore, if you wish to burn fat, you will be more successful in achieving your goals by adopting a consistent, low-intensity training program.

Protein

Protein is essential for growth and development. It is a component of hormones, antibodies, enzymes, and tissues. Protein is also essential in the repair of cells, including muscle cells. The proteins that make up the human body are not obtained directly from the diet. Rather, dietary protein is broken down into its constituent *amino acids*, which the body then uses to build the specific proteins it needs. Thus, amino acids rather than protein are the essential nutrients.

Of the twenty amino acids that your body uses to make protein, eleven are designated *nonessential* because they can be produced by your body from other amino acids, and do not need to be obtained from your diet. Your body cannot synthesize the nine *essential* amino acids, however. These must be broken down from the protein that you consume in your diet. All of the essential amino acids must be present in order for your body to build or repair muscle.

The way your body uses protein during and after exercise is much more complex than the way it uses carbohydrate or fat for energy. In the hours following exercise, your body begins to build structural proteins from amino acids for muscle repair and growth, remodeling the tissues that you need for performance. This is just one reason why paying careful attention to nutrition for complete recovery should be an important part of your training program.

Again, exercise intensity and duration are important factors in determining which of the nutrient fuels will be burned to energize your body. Low- to moderate-intensity exercise of long duration demands large quantities of fuel—often more than your carbohydrate and fat reserves can provide effectively. Therefore, your body begins to utilize structural and functional proteins during long-term aerobic exercise. Short-duration, high-intensity exercise, on the other hand, uses primarily glucose, so that your protein reserves are spared.

THE CHEMISTRY OF ENERGY PRODUCTION

Your body can break nutrients down to produce energy in three possible ways. The ATP-CP pathway and the glycolysis pathway are both forms of *anaerobic metabolism,* meaning that they do not require oxygen to generate ATP. Neither of these systems can use fat or protein directly as a fuel source, and therefore rely only on carbohydrate to produce energy. Anaerobic metabolism provides energy for high-intensity exercise such as sprinting down a basketball court or running 400 meters on a track. This energy is limited, however, lasting approximately ten seconds in duration for the ATP-CP pathway to several minutes in duration for glycolysis. In addition, glycolysis generates lactic acid as a byproduct. As lactic acid builds up, it slows down the ability of individual cells to produce energy, leading to muscle fatigue.

Aerobic metabolism is called into play for activities that demand a continuous supply of energy over a longer period of time, such as cross-country skiing, road cycling, swimming, and distance running. The aerobic pathway is advantageous for these types of activities because it produces a great deal more energy than anaerobic metabolism without generating lactic acid as a byproduct.

The ATP-CP Pathway

Your body uses the ATP-CP pathway to provide energy in situations requiring immediate, high-intensity actions. Because there is only enough adenosine triphosphate (ATP) stored in your body to last for five to ten seconds of intense exercise, ATP is continually synthesized to provide energy for your muscles to function.

Adenosine triphosphate is composed of three phosphate groups attached to an adenosine molecule by a chemical bond. The bond that connects the second and third phosphate groups is not very strong, so it is easily broken. When this occurs, a great deal of energy is released—energy that your body can then use for movement. (See Figure 2.1 on page 20.)

When the third phosphate group is removed from ATP the remaining molecule is *adenosine diphosphate,* or ADP. This molecule can be regenerated into ATP with the help of *creatine phosphate* (CP), which acts as a phosphate storage site within your muscles. CP donates a phosphate group to ADP, creating a new molecule of ATP.

The ATP-CP cycle can continue indefinitely—as long as

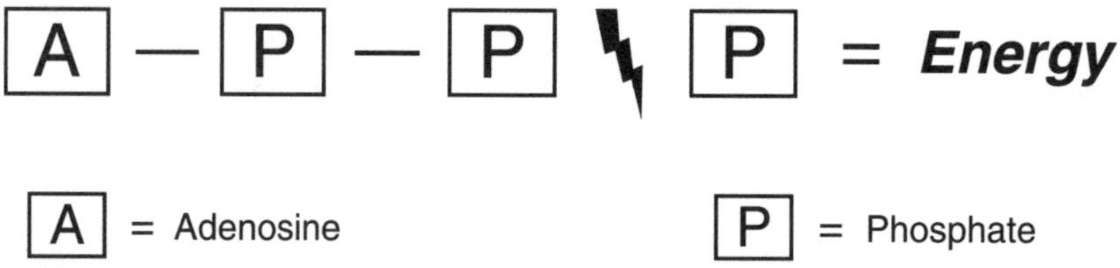

$$\boxed{A} - \boxed{P} - \boxed{P} \; \text{\Lightning} \; \boxed{P} = \textit{Energy}$$

$\boxed{A}$ = Adenosine $\boxed{P}$ = Phosphate

Figure 2.1. The release of energy from ATP

there's an adequate supply of creatine phosphate. When your CP reserves run low, however, your body begins to produce energy through the glycolysis pathway.

The Glycolysis Pathway

Like the ATP-CP pathway, glycolysis can occur without the presence of oxygen. In this energy pathway, stored glycogen—which is basically a long string of glucose molecules—is broken down into its glucose components. Through glycolysis, each molecule of glucose is split, and energy is released.

Glycolysis releases more energy than the ATP-CP pathway, so it is put into action when you engage in exercise that lasts from ten seconds to several minutes. But there is a disadvantage, because when there is an inadequate supply of oxygen, the glycolysis pathway produces *lactic acid* as a byproduct. For a time, lactic acid is quickly carried away from the muscles and returned to the liver, heart, and inactive muscles, where it is converted back into glucose. But blood and muscle concentrations begin to rise when lactic acid production proceeds at a faster pace than the speed with which it can be removed. When this occurs, you experience a burning sensation in your muscles. With a reduction in exercise intensity or a break from activity, however, the pain of lactic-acid buildup generally dissipates within twenty to thirty minutes.

The Aerobic Pathway

During short-duration, high-intensity exercise, your muscles rely primarily on the ATP-CP and glycolysis pathways to produce energy. After two to three minutes, the aerobic pathway becomes the principal energy pathway, as your body begins to use oxygen to burn nutrients for energy. An important difference between the anaerobic and aerobic pathways concerns the types of nutrients that can be used to produce energy. As you can see in Figure 2.2, the aerobic pathway uses fatty acids and amino acids in addition to glucose for energy.

Nature has established a metabolic priority system that determines when each nutrient will be mobilized as a fuel source. This system is based on the availability and efficiency with which your muscle cells can use the three nutrients. Glucose is the only fuel that can be used to produce energy in the anaerobic pathways, so it is used when there is insufficient oxygen for aerobic metabolism. Glycogen, the storage form of glucose, is found mostly in muscle and liver cells, so it can be mobilized rapidly and used as an immediate source of fuel.

When your body shifts over to the aerobic pathway for energy production, fat is used in addition to glucose for

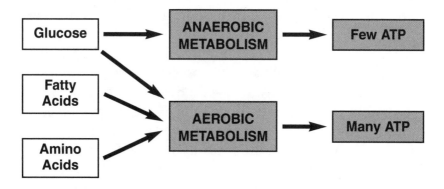

Figure 2.2. Energy production in the anaerobic and aerobic pathways

energy. Because fat is stored mostly in the adipose tissues of the body, it is not as easily accessible as carbohydrate—it is first broken down into fatty acids before being transported to the working muscles by the blood. Your body tends to spare protein as an energy source because of its numerous other functions in the body. As explained earlier in the chapter, protein is used primarily to build and repair tissues. Therefore, protein is used only as other fuels sources begin to run low.

HOW ENDURANCE TRAINING ALTERS ENERGY PRODUCTION

Endurance training brings about a number of adaptive changes in your body. First, it increases the number of capillaries surrounding each muscle cell—sometimes by up to 40 percent. More of these small blood vessels provide for a greater exchange of oxygen and vital nutrients between the blood and the working muscle cells. Training also increases the number of red blood cells that deliver oxygen to the muscle cells. Combined, these changes help to make aerobic energy production more efficient.

Once oxygen is delivered to the cell membrane, it is transported within the cell by *myoglobin*. Myoglobin content in skeletal muscle increases significantly following endurance training. This increase in myoglobin, however, occurs only within the muscles involved in the training and does not take place in less active muscles. Myoglobin's main function is to deliver oxygen from the cell membrane to the sites of energy production called *mitochondria*.

Aerobic energy production is the exclusive responsibility of the mitochondria. These tiny, sack-like structures within your cells combine carbohydrate, fat, and protein with oxygen to produce chemical energy in the form of ATP. Within the mitochondria, the breakdown of fuels and the ultimate production of ATP depends upon the action of protein molecules called *enzymes*. These proteins initiate or speed chemical reactions in the body. Regular endurance training increases the number of enzymes in the mitochondria, allowing for a faster conversion of nutrient fuels into ATP. This increases in the amount of energy produced in your muscle cells—and more energy means that you are able to exercise longer and at a higher intensity than are lesser-trained athletes.

Muscle biopsy studies have shown that there are two major changes associated with mitochondrial energy production following endurance training: an increase in the number and the size of the mitochondria. Research has shown a progressive weekly increase of approximately 5 percent in the number of muscle mitochondria over a six-month period of endurance training. These steady but gradual changes in mitochondria suggest that the structural improvements associated with endurance training may take months and perhaps years to fully develop.

All individuals who train with the same duration and intensity will show similar adaptations in muscle, regardless of their innate talents. Despite the variety of changes that occur in the muscles during training, the adaptations that elite athletes experience are very similar to those seen in athletes who train for local races without ever winning a gold medal. Champions are born with "good genes" but they still have to put in the long hours of training to achieve their full potential.

CONCLUSION

In order for your muscles to carry out the essential processes involved in contraction, they must be able to generate energy from the macronutrients that you consume in the form of food and nutritional supplements. Through digestion and metabolism, carbohydrate, fat, and protein are broken down into smaller molecules of glucose, fatty acids, and amino acids, respectively. Your body "burns" these fuels—with or without oxygen—to generate energy in the form of ATP for muscle contraction.

Endurance training enhances the environment for energy production by increasing the amount of ATP produced in your muscles. But training alone does not guarantee optimal performance. Chapter 3 examines the six factors that can cause muscle fatigue, and will guide you in learning to recognize and avoid them.

3.

WHAT CAUSES
MUSCLE FATIGUE?

As a sports scientist, I've had the opportunity to participate in a great deal of research concerning the causes of "hitting the wall." Any athlete who has experienced this extreme muscle fatigue knows that it can make crossing the finish line a difficult—if not impossible—goal to achieve. Numerous studies have pointed to dehydration and carbohydrate depletion as the causes of exercise-induced fatigue. To some extent, this is true.

Today, endurance athletes know that they can prolong activity by practicing carbohydrate loading prior to extended training sessions or long competitive events. They are also aware of the importance of drinking fluids before and during exercise to prevent dehydration and heat-related illness. However, many athletes—professional or otherwise—do not know the full extent of what causes muscle fatigue. This chapter explores several other factors that contribute to fatigue, including depletion of muscle fuels, low blood glucose, increased lactic-acid levels, and central fatigue.

DEHYDRATION

As discussed in Chapter 2, water is an essential macronutrient in every function of the body. During exercise, it's
important to make sure that you drink water because of
its vital role in cardiovascular function and temperature
regulation.

When you exercise, your body loses water through
sweating and evaporation. Sweat is your body's coolant.
During an intense workout, your muscles generate heat,
which is carried by your blood through capillaries near the
surface of your skin. Your sweat glands release perspiration that evaporates, cooling the skin and the blood just
underneath. Cooled blood then flows back to cool your
body's core.

Sweating is therefore an essential mechanism for regu-
lating body temperature. However, when your body loses
water it limits the capacity of your blood to carry vital
nutrients, such as glucose, fatty acids, and oxygen, to
working muscles. The capacity of the blood to remove
the byproducts of metabolism, including carbon dioxide
and lactic acid, is compromised as well. The result is an
increased demand on the circulatory system, which is
approximately 70-percent water.

I have seen some cyclists set out for a fifty- to seventy-
five-mile ride with only two small water bottles. On a hot
day, the weight lost through sweat may be as much as 5 to
6 pounds. Even if a rider drinks both bicycle-style bottles,
equaling about 40 ounces of water, he or she will replace
only two and a half pounds of lost fluid. In such cases,
dehydration is inevitable. At the very least, this limits the
cyclist's athletic performance. More seriously, it puts the
athlete in jeopardy of experiencing heat-related illness and
even circulatory collapse.

Even a slight dehydration—as little as 2 percent of your
body weight—can impair athletic performance. Athletes

must drink fluids to combat the sweat loss that naturally accompanies vigorous exercise. Although it may be impossible to offset all of the water lost through sweating, even partial replacement can minimize the risk of overheating.

Pure water is acceptable for replacing fluids, but drinking water is not the best way to rehydrate during and after exercise. To restore the body fluids that you sweat out during exercise, you should consume a beverage that contains agents such as glucose and sodium, two ingredients found in most sports or energy drinks. Glucose and sodium help maintain blood volume, and aid the absorption of water into your body. These two ingredients also increase thirst, which will prompt you to continue drinking—and the more you drink, the more completely you'll restore lost body fluids.

OVERHEATING

An athlete's temperature, normally about 98.6°F, may increase to 104°F or more during intense exercise. As explained earlier in the chapter, the circulatory system transports the heat generated by muscles to the skin to be dissipated. While a certain percentage of blood is used to regulate body temperature, large quantities of blood are still required to meet the energy and metabolic needs of working muscles. These demands may overtax the circulatory system, resulting in an inadequate removal of body heat and a corresponding rise in the athlete's body temperature.

Even in mild weather you can run the risk of overheating. The threat becomes more severe when weather conditions are hot and humid. Sweat doesn't evaporate well in this sort of climate because the surrounding air is already saturated with water. Without the cooling effects of sweat evaporation, your body is unable to maintain a constant body temperature that's within normal limits. If you con-

Do Men Perspire
More Than Women?

Some studies have suggested that women do not run as great a risk as men of becoming too dehydrated during exercise. The idea is that women sweat more efficiently than men, and therefore lose less fluid. In a study to see if women really do have an edge in hot, humid weather, twelve runners—six female and six male—ran twenty-five miles in the hot Georgia sun. Temperatures during the run varied from 77 to 90°F, and relative humidity averaged a sauna-like 70 to 80 percent.

These twelve volunteers were all in great shape. The men had been running an average of fifty-two miles per week, while the women ran an average of fifty-three miles. The men completed the twenty-five miles in an average of 173.5 minutes, while the women required about 183.8 minutes. Despite the time differences, all of the men and women were actually running at about 75 percent of maximum effort.

tinue to exercise in this state, you will increase your chances of suffering from heat exhaustion.

The hazards of exercising in hot, humid conditions were made abundantly clear at the 1996 Olympic Games in Atlanta, Georgia. A cycling road race was held on a day when temperatures exceeded 85°F, in unfavorable conditions of high humidity and no cloud cover. Several athletes from New Zealand and Denmark dropped out, and a Swedish rider collapsed after the finish and had to be hospitalized. The symptoms that these athletes developed undeniably indicated heat exhaustion. (See Table 3.1 on page 30.)

Just before they set out on their run, all twelve runners drank 14 ounces of a beverage containing carbohydrate and electrolytes. During the run, the men each drank approximately 29 ounces of fluid, while the women drank about 23 ounces each. Interestingly enough, sweat rates for the men turned out to be far higher. Men sweated out 1.70 liters of water per hour, and totaled about 3.80 liters during the run. Women, on the other hand, lost only about 1.25 liters each hour, totaling 2.65 liters of fluid. Thus, the average male runner lost about a liter more of water than the average female during the twenty-five-mile run. Women also finished the run with lower body temperatures, lost less blood-plasma volume, and maintained better levels of electrolytes in their blood.

This doesn't mean that women should be less concerned about replacing fluids when running on hot, humid days, however. The differences between the sexes weren't great enough to warrant totally different guidelines for women. In the heat, it's usually best to be on the safe side and drink plenty of fluids.

Research has proven that athletes involved in endurance sports other than distance cycling experience similar risks for overheating. In the 1970s, studies conducted by Dr. David Costill at the Human Performance Laboratory at Ball State University found that athletes who drank fluids during a two-hour run lowered their body temperatures by 2 degrees, when compared with athletes who did not rehydrate. Without fluid intake, one athlete's temperature reached 105.5°F during exercise, but it only reached 103.6°F when he drank fluids. Body temperature above 104.5°F causes great physical and mental stress, and is extremely dangerous. Therefore, fluid replacement is absolutely critical during training or competition—especially on a hot day.

If you're preparing for competition, it's wise to drink extra fluids in the few days before you compete, because drinking ensures maximum tissue hydration at the start of an event. You should also drink fluids before and at frequent intervals during a long event, in order to keep your body temperature at safe levels.

DEPLETION OF MUSCLE FUELS

During intense short-term exercise, fatigue can result from depletion of muscle glycogen. As explained in Chapter 2, this is because glucose is the only fuel source that your muscles use to generate energy through the anaerobic pathways, which last from ten seconds to several minutes in duration. During long-term exercise, the aerobic pathway kicks in for energy production. Fatty acids and amino acids are burned in addition to glucose as fuel for aerobic metabolism, providing a wider range of energy resources.

Studies have shown, however, that glycogen depletion contributes to muscle fatigue even during long-term exercise. When subjects exercised to exhaustion at 80 percent of

Table 3.1. Symptoms of Overheating

Body Temperature	Symptoms
101–104°F	Muscle weakness Fatigue
104–105°F	Disorientation Severe muscle weakness Loss of balance
Above 105°F	Diminished sweating Loss of consciousness

their maximum capacity, the glycogen content of their muscles dropped to near zero in about ninety minutes. Endurance was increased when glycogen storage capacity in the muscles was enhanced through carbohydrate loading. (For a detailed discussion of carbohydrate loading, see Chapter 12.) This suggests that your muscles' initial glycogen content plays an important role in exercise performance. Because glycogen is a crucial fuel for energy production, your muscle cells attempt to conserve glycogen during extended exercise. As you continue to exercise, fat stores are mobilized and fatty acids are used in approximately equal amounts as glycogen to provide energy. Finally, protein begins to provide a greater percentage of energy.

If you exercise primarily to burn fat, you'll be happy to know that it's possible to train your muscles to become more efficient in using fat as a fuel source by completing several extended training sessions, each lasting more than two hours. This method stimulates the enzymes responsible for the conversion of stored fat into energy, which will enable you to burn a higher percentage of fat and conserve glycogen for more strenuous efforts. The increased capacity of trained athletes to use fat, and the tendency of their muscles to release more fatty acids from fat tissue, suggests that training can shift the proportion of energy produced through the metabolism of fat.

LOW BLOOD GLUCOSE

In addition to providing necessary energy for muscle contraction, glucose is a vital source of energy for the brain and nervous system. Although fatty acids and amino acids can be used for voluntary muscle movement, glucose is the only fuel that can be used in sufficient amounts for nervous system function. In fact, 50 to 60 percent of the glucose supplied by the liver is used strictly for brain and nervous system function.

During the early phase of exercise, most of the energy supplied by carbohydrate comes from muscle glycogen. As exercise continues and muscle glycogen stores run low, glycogen contributes less and less as a source of energy. Figure 3.1 shows the proportions of nutrient fuels that are used during exercise. After about two hours of endurance exercise, muscle glycogen stores decrease rapidly. This reduced reliance on muscle glycogen is balanced by an increased reliance on blood glucose for fuel.

After two to three hours of exercise, the majority of carbohydrate energy appears to be derived from glucose, which is transported from circulating blood into the exercising muscles. This causes blood glucose to decline to relatively low levels. The liver, which has been supplying some amount of glucose from its glycogen stores, reduces its output due to depletion of liver glycogen. Fatigue occurs because there is not enough blood glucose available to compensate for the depleted muscle glycogen.

Studies by Christensen and Hansen in the 1960s demonstrated that subjects who exercised to exhaustion and then consumed 200 grams of glucose extended performance by one hour. In this experiment, the nervous system's

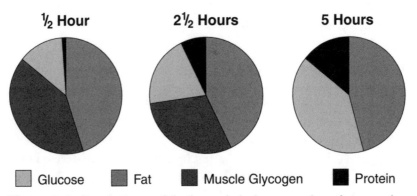

Figure 3.1. Proportions of fuel used during exercise. As exercise duration increases, your body relies less on muscle glycogen, and more on blood glucose, fat, and protein.

fuel had been depleted and restored. These results suggest that exhaustion may sometimes be a phenomenon of the central nervous system and not only the result of depleted muscle fuel stores.

As a long race continues, many athletes consume sports drinks, carbohydrate gels, and sports bars in an attempt to avoid fatigue. The use of these products helps athletes to keep blood glucose levels elevated to maintain central nervous system function, in addition to providing carbohydrate to working muscles. Research by Edward Coyle, Ph.D., from the University of Texas has shown that, during exercise, athletes are capable of absorbing up to 80 grams of carbohydrate per hour. This can delay fatigue by as much as thirty to sixty minutes, because the working muscles can rely primarily on blood glucose for energy.

INCREASED LACTIC-ACID LEVELS

Lactic acid is a byproduct of anaerobic metabolism that cannot be used effectively by your working muscles. Instead, lactic acid diffuses into your bloodstream to be transported to your heart, liver, and non-working muscles, where it is converted back into glucose. As you begin to exercise harder, more lactic acid builds up in your muscles, and must be removed by your blood. The lactic-acid level of your blood, therefore, continues to increase as exercise intensity increases. If this level of intensity is maintained, you will soon reach your *lactate threshold*, defined as the point at which the level of lactic acid in your blood is greater than your body can metabolize. Figure 3.2 on page 34 illustrates how blood lactate concentration increases with an increase in exercise intensity.

Most coaches and scientists consider the lactate threshold to be an excellent indicator of an athlete's potential for endurance performance. The ability to exercise at a high intensity without accumulating lactic acid is very benefi-

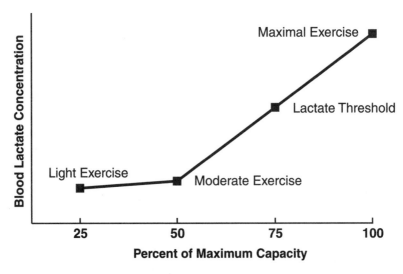

Figure 3.2. Blood lactate concentration during exercise. As exercise intensity increases, the lactic-acid level in the blood also increases.

cial. Generally, in two athletes with similar oxygen uptakes, the athlete with the higher lactate threshold will perform better in endurance activities. Laboratory and field experiments suggest that training can alter the amount of lactic acid produced and tolerated by athletes. This adaptation probably results from an increased efficiency of aerobic metabolism, as well as an increase in the number of capillaries that deliver oxygen to the muscles.

Lactic-acid buildup causes burning pain and muscle fatigue if it is not removed quickly from the muscles. Although lactic acid can be tolerated for short periods of time, your muscles should be allowed to relax at every opportunity. This allows your bloodstream to carry the lactic acid away, and to supply your tissues with oxygen for aerobic metabolism.

CENTRAL FATIGUE

In addition to focusing on the causes of muscle fatigue,

recent research has also centered on mental fatigue during exercise. This is commonly called *central fatigue* because it results from impaired function of the central nervous system. Although central fatigue does not affect your muscles directly, it can reduce your capacity to perform.

Dr. Eric Newsholme of Oxford University has uncovered a correlation between levels of the amino acid *tryptophan* in the brain and the degree of mental fatigue. When tryptophan enters the brain, it can depress the central nervous system, causing sleepiness and fatigue. Normally, there are sufficient amounts of the branched-chain amino acids (BCAAs) *leucine, isolucine,* and *valine* in the blood to regulate the entry of tryptophan into the brain. During long-term exercise, however, muscle cells begin to use greater amounts of amino acids for energy. Your body prefers to use the BCAAs for energy because they can actually take the place of glucose in energy pathways. As your muscles begin to use the BCAAs for energy, the level of BCAAs drops, which allows for the entry of tryptophan into the brain, causing mental fatigue.

Research suggests that regular supplementation with branched-chain amino acids can prevent or forestall central fatigue by preventing tryptophan from entering the brain. Supplementation before and during exercise has been proven to increase performance during a soccer game and after a 30-kilometer race. Likewise, in a study of 193 marathoners, branched-chain amino acid supplementation improved performance in the slower runners. Additional research is being conducted on this fascinating area of study.

CONCLUSION

Today, sports scientists and nutritionists know that dehydration and carbohydrate depletion are not the only two factors that cause fatigue. Factors such as elevated lactic-acid levels and central fatigue also contribute to exhaustion. By making sure that you're properly hydrated before and during exercise, and by consuming enough of the nutrients that your body needs to fuel activity, you can greatly reduce your chances of hitting the wall.

Clearly, minimizing fatigue is one step toward maximizing performance. Rebuilding and repairing muscle tissue is another important factor in the strength and endurance equation. Before we can discuss how your muscles recover and develop after exercise, however, we have to look at the kinds of muscle damage that are caused by exercise. Just what are your muscles recovering from?

4.

WHAT CAUSES
MUSCLE SORENESS?

There will be times when your muscles are stiff and sore the day after an intense training session no matter what your level of fitness or athletic skill is. You may wonder how your body could let you down like this—especially if you've already put so much time and effort into your exercise program. Whatever you did, you did too much. Now it's the day after and you have an athletic hangover. Despite the pain, you may choose to stick to your training schedule, without decreasing intensity or duration. Perhaps you've taken to heart the "no pain, no gain" theory of training, and you actually find encouragement in your aching muscles. But what you and many other dedicated athletes don't know, and should be aware of, is that you're putting tremendous strain on your bodies—strain that could have long-term adverse effects on your physical and emotional health.

In the past, lactic-acid buildup was considered to be the cause of prolonged muscle fatigue and discomfort. However, lactic acid is completely washed out of the muscles within the sixty minutes after your exercise session. Since muscle soreness does not make itself known until twenty-four to thirty-six hours later, it's been necessary to seek out other explanations.

MECHANICAL DAMAGE

Current scientific research points to muscle damage as the primary cause of muscle soreness. When you strain your muscles, you produce localized damage such as microscopic tears to muscle fiber membranes and protein filaments. Over the twenty-four hours following strenuous exercise, the damaged muscles become swollen and sore. In addition, there is increased blood flow to the muscles, which causes the muscle tissues to swell. Muscle nerves perceive this abnormal state and send pain messages to your brain as soon as you try to move the morning after overexertion. By moving sore muscles, you increase circulation, which brings protein and other nutrients to muscles that need to be repaired. Moving stiff and sore muscles also helps to reduce swelling. This gradually begins to restore them to a normal state. However, you will not be able to exercise to your full potential because the damaged muscles have lost some strength.

Scientists have identified a biochemical marker called *creatine phosphokinase* (CPK) that is an excellent measure of muscle damage. CPK is an enzyme used in metabolism that is found mainly in the cells of skeletal and heart muscle. When skeletal muscle is damaged due to a muscle tear or from overuse, CPK begins to leak out of the muscles' cells, and blood levels of CPK rise within the hour. Research suggests that the rise in CPK is proportionate to the amount of skeletal muscle damage.

Typical short-term treatments for sore muscles include stretching, massage, topical application of sports balms or creams, submersion in a hot tub, or a session in the sauna. Some athletes also turn to aspirin and anti-inflammatory medication to reduce pain and inflammation. The real cure for muscle soreness, however, is prevention. The key is to gradually increase the difficulty and duration of your training program. Also, remember to stretch before and after every exercise session, and to warm up and cool down properly. You will find guidelines for stretching in Chapter 15.

Remember that activities such as cycling, running, and swimming, and stop-and-go sports such as basketball, use certain muscles that are not used regularly in daily life. The principle of specificity of training must be kept in mind, and your muscles, tendons, and ligaments should be allowed to adapt to a particular sport, activity, or movement pattern over a period of time.

As we grow older, our muscles and their surrounding tissues lose elasticity, so we feel soreness and tightness more quickly than we did in high school. Individuals who stay in shape into their thirties and forties should be able to exercise with minimal muscle soreness. After a very hard day of aerobic exercise or an intense session in the weight room, however, their muscles may feel somewhat stiff. Again, thorough warm-up and cool-down periods that include stretching should minimize this discomfort.

FREE-RADICAL DAMAGE

Recently, a great deal of research has focused on the link between free-radical formation and muscle damage. Free radicals are continuously formed as a normal consequence of body processes, and are also caused by environmental factors such as air pollution and radiation. You may be surprised to find out, however, that exercise has been associated with the formation of free radicals, as well. So what are these molecules, and how are they a threat to you, the health-conscious athlete?

All of your body's cells are made up of atoms that, in turn, contain paired particles called *electrons*. When every electron in an atom is paired with another electron, the atom is said to be stable. A *free radical* is an atom or a group of atoms (a molecule) that is short one electron, and is considered to be highly unstable. In order to restabilize itself, the free radical will actively seek out and steal an electron from another part of the cell. Free radicals are also known as *oxidants* because oxygen is usually the atom that loses an electron and then snatches other molecules' electrons. Therefore, free-radical damage is also known as *oxidative stress*.

There is evidence that long-term aerobic activity, including running, bicycling, and cross-country skiing, increases the production of these highly unstable molecules. Free radicals can damage muscle cell membranes and increase protein breakdown. They can also attack the walls of your muscle cells and mitochondria, and are at least partially to blame for muscle inflammation and soreness, which contribute to reduced endurance.

Research has shown that antioxidants may be vital components in reducing post-exercise muscle soreness. Antioxidants are vitamins and vitamin-like nutrients that can neutralize free radicals. Vitamins E and C are some of the better known antioxidants. These two nutrients are discussed individually in Chapter 8.

THE CORTISOL RESPONSE

Cortisol is a hormone that's released in response to all kinds of stress, including psychological, physical, and emotional stresses. Exercise places physical stress on your body, which stimulates the release of cortisol from small glands called *adrenal glands* attached to the top of each kidney. The primary role of cortisol is to help mobilize energy for the body. It does this by attacking muscle tissues directly, and increasing the rate at which protein in the muscles is broken down. In addition to this, cortisol impedes the entry of amino acids into muscle cells for protein synthesis, and instead helps to transport them to the liver to be used for energy. This is why individuals involved in strength training may experience a decrease in muscle mass if they do not take the necessary steps to reduce the release of cortisol and to rebuild muscle protein.

For a number of years, athletes have used anabolic (muscle-building) steroids to negate the effects of cortisol by helping the body to build itself back up. With steroid use, amino acids are taken up by the muscles at a higher rate to help repair some of the damage caused by cortisol when it extracts important nutrients for energy. However, the long-term use of anabolic steroids has been linked to the development of illnesses such as liver cancer and heart disease. In Chapter 9, we'll see how the R^4 system can help you blunt the rise of cortisol naturally.

CONCLUSION

Sore muscles are usually damaged muscles. As with any injury, sore muscles must be given time to heal. Keep in mind that the majority of muscle development occurs during the post-exercise recovery period. When you disregard pain and stiffness, you are actually doing more harm than good, because you are not giving your body time to recover from the mechanical and biochemical damage caused by exercise. And getting right back on the treadmill, so to speak, will only cause further damage to muscles that have already been weakened. These effects, coupled with physical discomfort, will make it impossible for you to exercise at peak capacity during subsequent training sessions.

Fortunately, research has proven that recovery can negate some of the physical effects of exercise. Chapter 5 examines the three critical phases of recovery during which energy stores are replenished and muscle damage is repaired. In doing so, it establishes the foundation for the R^4 System for Peak Performance.

5.

RECOVERY: YOUR KEY TO PEAK PERFORMANCE

Your ability to continue exercising day after day is limited by how quickly your muscles recover after exertion. Recovery ensures that your body returns to a normal, balanced state through the restoration of body fluids, replenishment of energy stores, and repair of damaged muscle tissues. In addition, your immune system, which is compromised by strenuous exercise, can be enhanced with adequate rest and careful attention to nutrition. By taking the proper steps to aid your body's recovery from exercise, you will increase your level of performance during training sessions or competitive events. More important, your overall health and strength will be improved.

THE THREE PHASES OF RECOVERY

Recovery from extended exercise is a complex process, but it can be broken down into three parts. The first phase of recovery, known as the rapid phase, occurs in the first thirty minutes after exercise. This is followed by the intermediate phase, which lasts up to two hours. The longer phase of recovery occurs during the remaining twenty hours before your next exercise session.

The Rapid Phase

The rapid phase of recovery begins when you finish your training session, and lasts for approximately thirty minutes. During this time, your body's metabolic rate slows and begins to return to pre-exercise levels. Your heart rate, respiratory rate, and body temperature start to return to their lower resting levels. Blood levels of certain hormones, such as cortisol and testosterone, which were elevated during exercise, begin to decrease. At the same time, your muscles start to replenish their stores of creatine phosphate and ATP, which were depleted to fuel activity. This is also the period during which your body removes excessive lactic acid that may have accumulated in your muscles. The majority of the lactic acid enters the bloodstream and circulates to the liver and inactive muscles, where it is reconverted into glucose.

The metabolic and physiological processes that occur during the rapid phase of recovery can be hastened by gentle exercise during the cool-down period. Exercising at 40 to 60 percent of maximum effort for five to ten minutes helps to keep your blood circulating at an increased rate. Keeping blood flow at a higher-than-normal rate during this phase aids in the removal of lactic acid from your muscles, and rapidly transports it to the appropriate sites for conversion.

The Intermediate Phase

The intermediate phase of recovery continues in the ninety minutes to two hours after exercise. During this time, your body begins the process of restoring fluid volumes, called *rehydration*. This is also the most critical period for the replenishment of muscle glycogen, in which the hormone insulin plays a vital role. Insulin facilitates the transport of glucose from your blood into your muscle cells. It also stimulates *glycogen synthase*, an enzyme in your muscle cells that is responsible for converting glucose into glycogen for storage.

Research conducted by Dr. John Ivy at the University of Texas at Austin's Exercise Physiology and Metabolism Laboratory has provided insight into why the intermediate phase is such a critical stage in the recovery process. Dr. Ivy discovered that muscle cells are most sensitive to insulin during this time. This means that when a sufficient source of carbohydrate is present, glycogen replenishment occurs at a faster rate. In fact, the speed of glycogen synthesis in the two hours following exercise is almost two to three times faster than normal.

In order to take full advantage of this increased insulin sensitivity, Ivy recommends drinking a carbohydrate-containing beverage such as a sports drink as soon after an event or training session as possible. If you don't consume a carbohydrate supplement during this period, you'll miss the period of maximum insulin sensitivity, and the rate of glycogen recovery will be significantly slowed. Thus, the longer you wait to replenish your glycogen stores, the longer it will take you to recover. As you will see in Chapter 6, consuming the proper ratio of carbohydrate and protein in your post-exercise meal or snack can increase your body's sensitivity to insulin during this critical phase, as well.

The Longer Phase

The longer phase of recovery spans the two to twenty hours following a workout. Carbohydrate replenishment continues in this interval, although at a lesser rate than during the first two hours following exercise. It's recommended that you consume 3 to 5 grams of carbohydrate per pound of your body weight during the hours between workouts. Most of your carbohydrate intake during this time should come from foods such as pasta, breads, and vegetables. These are *complex carbohydrates,* which consist of long chains of glucose that must first be broken down during digestion. This breakdown ensures a slow, steady supply of glycogen.

A crucial element in the long-term recovery process is muscle repair. During heavy exercise, the membranes of muscle fibers, the connective tissue surrounding them, and the actin and myosin filaments of your muscles are damaged. Less strenuous exercise also damages muscles, but to a lesser degree. Therefore, whether you engage in a moderate activity, such as jogging, or a more strenuous exercise like weightlifting, sprinting, or high-intensity running or cycling, your muscles require time and nutrients for repair. The long-term phase of recovery is the period in which muscles are repaired and adapt to exercise, which increases strength and endurance. The question, then, concerns how much "damage" you must do in order for your muscles to become stronger. Do you have to exercise to the point of muscle soreness?

"That's probably not necessary, because you can go in small steps and get the same types of changes," says William Evans, Ph.D., of the Nutrition, Metabolism, and Exercise Laboratory at the University of Arkansas for Medical Sciences in Little Rock. In fact, when you have extreme soreness and pain—the kind that gives you trouble jogging, moving your limbs, or lifting a heavy object—research shows that your strength is reduced, sometimes by as much as 25 percent. And the more you hurt, the longer it takes to recover your strength so that you can again exercise at your peak capacity.

The stresses of exercise also compromise your immune system, making you more susceptible to colds and infections. The intensity of your chosen activity, as well as your physical condition, influences the impact that exercise will have on your immune system, according to Dr. Evans. But, as you will see in Chapter 8, this damage can be minimized or even prevented.

THE DANGERS OF OVERTRAINING

In *The Lore of Running*, Dr. Tim Noakes gives examples of several nationally ranked athletes who exhibited symptoms of *overtraining syndrome*, or OTS. One athlete complained that he was lethargic and sleeping poorly. He also had less enthusiasm for training, and particularly for competition. He expressed concern that his legs felt "sore" and "heavy" and that the feelings had lasted for several training sessions. This athlete was obviously in need of complete rest from hard training.

The phenomena of overtraining are very real for the aerobic athlete. In training, it is a difficult—but essential—task to find your optimal training threshold and not to exceed the limits of your stress and adaptation capacities. Specific physiological and psychological changes are related to overtraining, which lead to a corresponding deterioration of athletic performance.

The symptoms of overtraining may be seen in an athlete who is eager to excel and begins to train frequently and intensely. At first, the athlete improves. After a while, however, his times stagnate and remain below his set goals. Anxious to pass the plateau, the athlete begins to train even harder. Instead of improving, his performance deteriorates and a sense of inadequacy and frustration develop. In addition to a decline in performance, there are corresponding changes in personality and behavior. The athlete gradually loses self-confidence, and suffers from chronic fatigue.

Are you worried that you or someone you know is overtraining? It's important to watch out for the following symptoms:

Physical Changes

- Constipation or diarrhea
- Fatigue
- Flu-like symptoms, including fever, chill, aches
- Gradual weight loss
- Heavy feeling in legs
- Inability to complete training
- Increased morning heart rate
- Lack of appetite
- Muscle soreness
- Swelling in lymph nodes

Emotional and Behavioral Changes

- Anxiety
- Depression
- Desire to quit training
- Inability to concentrate
- Irritability
- Loss of enthusiasm for training and competition
- Sleep disturbances

In the early 1980s, Dick Brown, then administrator and physiologist for the world-class running club Athletics West, conducted an experiment to try to identify warning signs of overtraining. He asked athletes to record several indicators in their training diaries, including morning body weight, morning heart rate, and amount of sleep. His research showed that if an athlete's morning heart rate is at least 10-percent higher than normal, if the athlete receives 10 percent less sleep than usual, or if the athlete's weight is down 3 percent or more, the athlete's body has not recovered from the previous hard workout. Therefore, to be on the safe side, you should cut back on your workout if you are abnormal in two indicators. Abnormal readings for all three indicators are a red flag, signaling that you should take the day off.

In order to ensure that you prevent the complications of overtraining before they occur, you should take the following measures into account:

- Use the nutritional principles of the R^4 System to make sure that you are maximizing recovery. These four principles are detailed in Part II.

- Sleep at least eight hours a night when you are engaged in a strenuous training program.

- Follow the guidelines presented in Chapters 11 and 12 to ensure that you are eating a balanced diet.

- Conduct at least eight to ten weeks of endurance work to build up a good base of conditioning.

- Gradually build up the quantity and quality of training, so that you are prepared both physically and mentally for an increased volume of training. Do not increase the frequency, duration, and intensity of training sessions too quickly.

- Try to nap for fifteen minutes to a half an hour before an afternoon workout.

- Make sure that the intensity of your training is individualized to your level of fitness and experience.

- Use a training diary to record morning pulse rate, morning body weight, sleep patterns, medical problems, and training difficulties.

Remember that rest and recovery are essential if you want your muscles to grow and develop. The use of rest days on a periodic basis will increase your strength and allow you to perform at your peak level when you do exercise.

CONCLUSION

Once strenuous training or competition has ended for the day, sufficient rest and careful nutritional management become essential for future performance. Recovery begins the moment that you cross the finish line, walk in from the field, or get down off your bike. During the post-exercise period, your muscles must receive essential nutrients to recover from mechanical damage in the form of swelling and microscopic tears; oxidative damage caused by unstable free radicals; and tissue degradation due to the release of cortisol in response to exercise stress.

In these first few chapters, we have reviewed the physical structure of skeletal muscles, and how they function, or contract, to generate movement. You have also learned about the biochemistry behind muscle function—namely, the anaerobic and aerobic pathways in which the nutrient fuels, carbohydrate, fat, and protein are used to generate energy for movement. And now that you know the story behind why athletes experience muscle fatigue and soreness, and how the human body is equipped to recover, we are ready to move on to the specifics of the R^4 System. Part II examines, in detail, the steps that you should take in order to optimize your recovery.

PART II

THE R^4 SYSTEM FOR PEAK PERFORMANCE

In the past, you may have experienced days when you simply couldn't meet your training goals, no matter how hard you pushed yourself. Whether you were still aching from your previous workout, thwarted by a muscle cramp, or just plain exhausted, you simply weren't able to exercise at peak capacity. In such cases, what was your remedy for muscle soreness and fatigue? Did you take a day off from training, try painkillers, or use sports balms? Believe it or not, exercise-induced fatigue and soreness are not entirely inevitable. The truth is that you can, to some extent, avoid these unpleasant consequences.

Part II will guide you in maximizing your recovery with targeted nutrition. Each of the principles of the R^4 System is discussed individually in the following pages, so that you can learn how to restore fluids and electrolytes; replenish glycogen rapidly; reduce muscle stress; and rebuild muscle protein. By following the simple guidelines outlined in the next few chapters, you'll be able to extend your endurance and increase your muscle strength within days, in addition to minimizing muscle pain and boosting immunity. All of these benefits will enable you to perform at a higher level than you've ever thought possible.

6.

RESTORE FLUID AND ELECTROLYTES

Everybody knows that sweating is a natural consequence of exercise, and most people take some measures, during and after exercise, to replenish the fluids that they sweat out. The problem is that a lot of athletes aren't fully aware of the consequences of fluid loss during exercise. As we have already discussed, dehydration as little as 2 percent of body weight impairs performance. But diminished capacity for exercise isn't all there is to worry about. Because water is an essential nutrient for body temperature regulation and cardiovascular function, increased dehydration means increased risk of overheating and circulatory collapse. And, along with the water lost through sweating, your body also loses electrolytes, which are important for muscle contraction and relaxation.

Unfortunately, the human body is not well equipped to replenish the fluids that are lost through sweating and evaporation. We simply lack the capacity to take in and retain fluids at the rate with which they are lost during heavy exercise. This phenomenon is known as *involuntary dehydration*. The good news is that, by paying careful attention to what you drink and when you drink it, you can take steps to minimize dehydration and to restore electrolyte losses.

REHYDRATION

In order to understand how your body replenishes lost fluids, you should first understand what causes thirst. The thirst drive is dependent upon two factors: your body's blood volume, and the concentration of salts, or electrolytes, in your blood. When you lose fluids during exercise through sweating, your blood volume decreases. This results in a corresponding increase in the concentration of electrolytes in your blood, which stimulates thirst.

Drinking plain water is fine for events lasting less than sixty minutes. It's certainly better than not drinking fluids at all. However, when you drink plain water, you usually satisfy your thirst before you have actually consumed enough liquid to return blood volume and electrolyte concentrations to pre-exercise levels. In addition, rehydrating with plain water during exercise lasting for more than four hours can cause *hyponatremia,* or "water intoxication." This results from the dilution of sodium in the blood due to increased blood volume and excessive sodium losses in sweat. The symptoms of water intoxication include headache, nausea, muscle cramping, and lethargy.

Recent research has shown that your body absorbs more fluid when electrolytes such as sodium are added to water. In one study, six volunteers underwent two exposures to heat and then engaged in an exercise regimen that caused a mild dehydration, resulting in a 2- to 3-percent decrease in body weight. Each volunteer then drank either water or a water and sodium solution to replenish fluids. During the three-hour rehydration period, subjects who drank water alone restored 68 percent of the fluid they lost, while subjects who drank the sodium solution replaced 82 percent of their lost fluids.

What caused this marked difference? Subjects who drank plain water satisfied their thirst quickly for two reasons. First, water intake caused blood volume to increase, which eliminated the volume-dependent element of thirst. Second, plain water diluted sodium in the blood, resulting in a decrease in sodium concentration within 15 minutes. In this case, the body "shuts off" thirst to keep sodium concentrations within healthy limits. Thus, the dilution of sodium eliminated the salt-dependent element of the thirst drive.

On the other hand, sodium concentration remained significantly higher in subjects who drank water with added sodium. The addition of sodium to water helped to maintain the salt-dependent factor of the thirst drive, prompting the volunteers to continue drinking. This led to a more complete restoration of body fluids within the three-hour recovery period.

So how do you know if your sports drink is a good rehydration beverage? For a sports drink to be effective, it must contain at least 75 milligrams of sodium for every 8 ounces of fluid. This small amount of sodium in sports drinks helps maintain or restore the body's fluid and electrolyte balance. In addition, added sodium improves the flavor of the product, which encourages the athlete to drink more of it.

According to an American College of Sports Medicine consensus conference, carbohydrate should be an ingredient in rehydration drinks in addition to electrolytes. Research has shown that carbohydrate and sodium work together to increase water absorption in the intestinal wall. Carbohydrate's component glucose molecules stimulate sodium absorption, and sodium, in turn, is necessary for glucose absorption. When these two substances are absorbed by the intestines, they tend to pull water with them, thus facilitating the absorption of water from the intestines into the bloodstream.

ELECTROLYTE REPLACEMENT

Electrolytes such as sodium, chloride, potassium, and

magnesium are necessary elements for muscle contraction and relaxation. In addition, electrolytes help maintain your body's fluid balance. During exercise, your body loses some amount of these minerals with water through sweating. Because electrolytes are found in blood plasma and muscle tissues in varying concentrations, measured in milliequivalents per liter, or mEq/L, the concentrations lost through sweat vary, as well. (See Table 6.1 on page 57.)

Whereas drinking pure water to quench your thirst quickly reduces the drive for additional fluid consumption, the addition of electrolytes leads to a more complete restoration of body water content. This is because electrolytes are salts, so they help maintain the salt-dependent element of thirst. This leads to more effective rehydration and regulates your body temperature and cardiovascular function. Figure 6.1 summarizes this principle.

Sodium and Chloride

Sodium and chloride are electrolytes that help maintain the

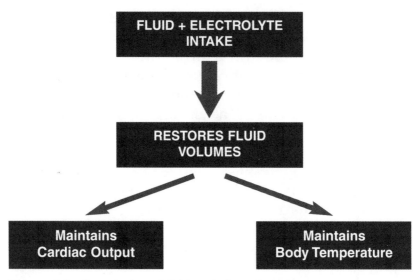

Figure 6.1. Restoration of fluid and electrolytes

Table 6.1. Electrolyte Concentrations in Blood Plasma, Muscle Tissues, and Sweat

	Sodium (mEq/L)	Chloride (mEq/L)	Potassium (mEq/L)	Magnesium (mEq/L)
Blood Plasma	140	100	4	1.5
Muscle Tissues	9	5	160	30
Sweat	40–60	30–50	4–5	1.5–5

volume and balance of all the fluids outside your body's cells, such as blood. Sodium plays a particularly important role because it helps transport nutrients into cells, so they can be used for energy production, as well as tissue growth and repair. In addition, sodium functions in muscle contraction and nerve impulse transmission.

The concentration of sodium and chloride lost in sweat is about one-third the concentration found in the plasma of your blood. Therefore, if you lose 9 pounds of sweat during a long race or training session, the electrolyte losses would be roughly 5 to 6 percent of your body's total sodium-chloride content.

Sodium and chloride are found in most foods, and can be easily obtained through a balanced diet. Therefore, sodium or chloride deficiency generally occurs because of severe dehydration, during long periods of exercise without proper fluid or electrolyte replenishment. The side effects include reduced performance, dizziness, and fainting.

Potassium

Potassium is necessary for nerve transmission, muscle contraction, and glycogen formation. It also aids in maintaining cardiovascular system function. Whereas sodium and chloride are highly concentrated in the fluids outside of your cells, the concentration of potassium in the fluid within your cells is almost forty times greater than the concentration in your blood. Therefore, potassium losses, which result in a decrease of less than one percent through sweat, are not as great as sodium and chloride losses. It has been suggested, however, that this small percentage is enough to cause muscles to contract involuntarily, resulting in painful cramps that can stop you in your tracks. In addition, potassium losses can lead to heat intolerance.

Potassium is lost in a number of ways during and after exercise. Because potassium is stored together with glycogen in the muscle fibers, the breakdown of glycogen to supply energy to your muscles leads to an increased loss of potassium from the muscle cells. This results in a corresponding increase in the potassium concentration of your blood. After exercise, potassium is excreted in greater quantities in the urine.

To replenish the potassium loss resulting from exercise, try drinking a sports recovery drink that contains potassium. It's also wise to eat a balanced diet that includes foods high in potassium, such as dairy foods, bananas, oranges, kiwi fruit, potatoes, and tomato juice.

Because potassium is present in most foods, deficiency is rarely reported. Depletion is generally due to severe dehydration. A common cause of potassium depletion is prolonged use of diuretics, which promote potassium excretion by the kidneys. The symptoms of potassium deficiency are numerous, and include nausea, diminished reflex function, fluctuations in heartbeat, drowsiness, and muscular fatigue and weakness.

Magnesium

Magnesium is found in all of your body's cells, although it is primarily located in the bones, muscles, and soft tissues. It's a necessary element in over 300 enzyme reactions involving nerve transmission, muscle contraction, and especially ATP production.

Research has shown that increased physical activity can deplete the body's magnesium stores. In one study, twenty-six runners were found to have significantly lower levels of magnesium in their blood and urine after they completed a marathon. This could be because the body uses more magnesium during prolonged intense exercise. When magnesium levels fall below a critical point, performance suffers, and athletes run a greater risk of developing muscle cramps.

Low blood magnesium levels during exercise have also been cited as causes of muscle fatigue and irregular heartbeat. Magnesium deficiency can lead to dizziness, muscle weakness, irritability, and depression, as well. Based on this information, it's important to consume a sports drink that contains magnesium in order to replenish what is lost during exercise. Sufficient magnesium can also be obtained by eating a balanced diet, which includes such magnesium-rich foods such as apples, avocados, bananas, brown rice, dairy foods, garlic, green leafy vegetables, soybeans, and whole grains.

Several studies have shown that supplementing the diet with moderate amounts of magnesium is not only beneficial in avoiding depletion, but may also improve endurance and strength. In a study of untrained subjects, ranging from eighteen to twenty years of age, who underwent a seven-week training schedule, greater improvements in muscle strength were found among those who took 560 milligrams of magnesium daily compared to those who received a placebo. A *placebo* is a "dummy pill" that doesn't contain active ingredients.

WHAT CAUSES MUSCLE CRAMPS?

Perhaps the simplest way to describe a cramp is as an out-of-control muscle contraction, which locks the muscle in a painful and sustained spasm. Unlike a normal muscle contraction, you have no control over when or where a cramp may strike—and if you don't act quickly, it can put you in a great deal of pain.

The cause of cramps is elusive. Several theories exist, but the most common one is exercise-induced dehydration. When you exercise heavily, you can lose large quantities of water through perspiration. This water loss lowers blood volume, so there is less blood going to muscles to deliver oxygen, resulting in a muscle spasm. Another possible cause of cramps related to dehydration is electrolyte imbalance. The electrolytes sodium and potassium, together with calcium and magnesium, help regulate muscle relaxation and contraction. Because you may lose electrolytes through extreme sweating, dehydration can contribute to an electrolyte imbalance. If there's an imbalance of these nutrients, muscles may contract involuntarily.

Muscles that are overly fatigued or overworked are prone to cramps; thus people who are not well trained are more likely to suffer from them. Some people are naturally more susceptible, and this may be due to inherently low electrolyte and mineral levels. Cold weather also seems to precipitate cramps in some athletes. Other less common causes include diabetes and circulatory and neurological disorders. Therefore, if you experience persistent cramps, you should consult your doctor.

Regardless of the cause, the treatment for immediate relief of muscle cramps is the same in every case: gently stretch the muscle as best you can, and apply pressure to the muscle while stretching to help unlock the cramp. Gentle massage can also be beneficial. The importance of good warm-up and cool-down periods cannot be emphasized enough. Stretching thoroughly before and after your workout can stop cramps before they start. If painful muscle cramps habitually wake you up at night, also stretch

before going to bed. Guidelines for stretching are presented in Chapter 15. Fortunately, there are several other steps
that you can take to prevent cramps altogether.

First, keep in mind the role of dehydration in causing
cramps, and drink plenty of fluids to remain sufficiently
hydrated, especially if you're exercising outdoors or in a
hot and humid environment. Don't let thirst determine
when you should drink fluids—by the time you're thirsty,
you may already be 2- to 3-percent dehydrated. Because
satisfying your thirst does not necessarily mean that you
have satisfied your body's need for fluids, you should continue to replenish fluids, even if you think you're not
thirsty. Chances are, your body is!

Also remember that it's crucial to get adequate amounts
of nutrients such as sodium, potassium, calcium, and magnesium in your diet, because these minerals are responsible for proper muscle contraction and relaxation. Magnesium appears to be especially critical for triggering the
relaxation of tensed muscles. However, simply popping a
magnesium supplement is not the answer. In order to be
most effective, magnesium needs to be properly balanced
with calcium. A two-to-one ratio of magnesium to calcium
is thought by many experts to provide the ideal balance
of these important minerals for muscle relaxation. This
ratio should not be confused with the 2 to 1 ratio of calcium to magnesium that is necessary for healthy bones (see
Chapter 12). To help relieve muscle spasms and soreness, it
is recommended that you supplement with 800 milligrams
of magnesium and 400 milligrams of calcium.

Many athletes underestimate the effect that a change in
environment can have on their ability to exercise. It's
important that you acclimate slowly to weather changes.
Take about two weeks to adjust to hot- or cold-weather
temperature changes, and cut back slightly during season-
al transitions. This will allow your body to adjust with a
minimal amount of physical stress. If you are vacationing

in a dramatically different climate, take it easy on yourself both while on holiday and when you arrive home.

Finally, consider the types of medication that you take. Various drugs such as diuretics and bronchial dilators have been implicated as causes of muscle cramps for some people. If you suffer from cramps and take any kind of medication, consult your physician to see if this may be the cause.

PREVENTING DEHYDRATION

There are several steps that you can take in order to replenish water and electrolytes during and after exercise. You should use the following tips as a guide in preventing dehydration and heat-related illness—especially when you're training or competing in hot, humid weather.

❏ Water is a good source of replenishment for exercise lasting less than one hour. However, sports beverages, which are formulated to encourage continued consumption, and to replace carbohydrate and some protein, are more effective fluid replacements.

❏ Drink up to 12 ounces of a sports drink fifteen minutes before exercise or competition. This drink should provide sufficient amounts of electrolytes, as shown in Table 6.2 below. Continue to replenish fluids by drinking 4 to 8 ounces of your sports drink every ten to fifteen minutes during your event or training session.

Table 6.2. Adequate Ranges of Electrolytes Per Eight Ounces of Recovery Drink

Electrolyte	Amount	Electrolyte	Amount
Sodium	75–250 mg	Potassium	200–330 mg
Chloride	45–75 mg	Magnesium	100–400 mg

❑ If you perspire heavily, you may require electrolytes such as sodium, potassium, and magnesium in greater-than-normal quantities. By adding a little extra salt to foods, or drinking a quality sports beverage, you can replace some of the electrolytes that you lose through sweat.

❑ Avoid carbonated drinks when you're thirsty, because they can cause gastrointestinal distress. Gas can make you feel full, which prevents you from drinking enough to fully rehydrate.

❑ Weigh yourself each morning, and record your weight on a chart or in a training diary. If you are well hydrated, your weight should be about the same each morning. If you find that your weight is down, you should drink 16 ounces of fluids for every pound that you have lost in body weight.

❑ An ideal fluid replacement beverage should stimulate fluid absorption, maintain proper fluid balance in the body, and provide energy to working muscles. And of course, the drink should taste good, so you'll want to drink more of it.

Most important, remember that thirst is not always a good indicator of your body's need for fluids. Don't allow yourself to lose water weight and get into a state of chronic dehydration. In hot and humid weather, be sure to drink plenty of fluids between meals and in the evening, not just during and immediately following exercise.

CONCLUSION

Taking the proper steps to rehydrate will reduce the chances that you'll overtax your circulatory system, as well as your risk of developing heat-related illnesses—and this will dramatically increase your ability to exercise at peak performance during training sessions. An important factor in rehydration is adequate intake of electrolytes. The addition of these mineral salts to many sports drinks not only helps to ensure healthy muscle function, but also stimulates the thirst drive, and aids in the absorption of water by your body. Clearly, restoring fluids and electrolytes is critical during and after exercise not only for performance, but for your overall health.

7.

REPLENISH GLYCOGEN RAPIDLY

In addition to restoring your body's fluid and electrolyte balance after exercise, you need to begin replenishing your muscle glycogen stores. Because glycogen supplies energy in the form of glucose to keep your muscles working, restoring its quantities in the liver and muscles is an important factor in optimal recovery from exercise. How fast glycogen is manufactured and stored determines how quickly you will be ready to compete or train again at peak capacity. As you will see, stimulating insulin is the key to rapid and complete replenishment of depleted glycogen.

INSULIN: THE MASTER RECOVERY HORMONE

Insulin is a hormone released by the pancreas in response to carbohydrate consumption. One of its main functions is to help transport glucose into liver and muscle tissues, where it is stored as glycogen. Insulin also stimulates the enzyme glycogen synthase, which aids in manufacturing glycogen from glucose.

As you learned in Chapter 4, timing is key in replenishing muscle glycogen. Your muscle cells are most sensitive to insulin during the first two hours following exercise. Assuming that enough carbohydrate is available, elevated levels of insulin in the blood after exercise speed up the transport of glucose to your muscle cells, and this accelerates the rate of glycogen manufacture. After two hours, muscle cells become more resistant to insulin, and remain so for several hours.

Clinical studies have proven that athletes who consume carbohydrate within two hours after exercise are able to more completely restore their muscles' glycogen levels. Athletes who waited more than two hours to consume carbohydrate restored about 50-percent less muscle glycogen than did athletes who consumed carbohydrate during the period of maximum insulin sensitivity. The most striking results were observed in soccer players who drank high-carbohydrate beverages between successive games. The players who had taken in carbohydrate were able to cover more yards in the next game, compared with players who did not supplement with carbohydrate. The lesson here is very clear: If you do not consume carbohydrate immediately after exercise, you will not be able to fully restore your muscles' glycogen stores—and depleted energy stores mean less energy for training or competition the next day.

During my work with the U.S. Cycling Team, as Co-ordinator of Sport Sciences, I tested this concept by having a group of cyclists consume carbohydrate immediately after the end of a training session. I found that in their next training session, performance improved and the cyclists did not feel as if they worked as hard. Clearly, replenishing muscle glycogen is of the utmost importance for optimal performance.

ENHANCING THE INSULIN RESPONSE

Because insulin is essential in replenishing muscle glycogen after exercise, researchers have focused on enhancing insulin release during recovery. Studies have shown that protein, when combined with carbohydrate, almost doubles the insulin response and increases the rate of glycogen synthesis by 30 percent. So it seems logical that any sports drink containing protein in addition to carbohydrate would offer an advantage in recovery.

However, more is less in this case. Protein stimulates a substance called *cholecystokinin*, or CCK, which slows the rate of gastric emptying. This is the rate at which your stomach contents are emptied into the intestines. Therefore, too much protein, then, slows fluid and electrolyte replacement during recovery, because fluids must first leave the stomach and enter the intestines to be absorbed into the bloodstream. Delayed gastric emptying slows fluid absorption and, as a result, rehydration.

The challenge, then, is how to gain the benefits of supplemental protein while avoiding the negative effect on gastric emptying. You can achieve this by carefully balancing carbohydrate and protein according to a critical ratio, which I call the *optimum recovery ratio*, or OR^2. When the ratio of carbohydrate to protein is 4 to 1, the protein does not seem to interfere with rehydration. For instance, if you consume 56 grams of carbohydrate after exercise, you would want to supplement this with 14 grams of protein, according to the ratio, in order to enhance the insulin response without affecting the rate of gastric emptying.

Recently, John Ivy, Ph.D., of the University of Texas, conducted research on the effect of the amino acid *arginine* on post-exercise recovery. Arginine helps stimulate the pancreas to release insulin, and is also known to be important for muscle metabolism. Dr. Ivy studied the effects of carbohydrate supplements that contained arginine on the rate of muscle glycogen synthesis after exercise. Carbohydrate-arginine supplementation increased muscle-glycogen replenishment by 35 percent more than carbohydrate

alone. Ivy concluded that arginine, when added to carbohydrate, makes more glucose available for glycogen production. It produces this effect by increasing the use of fat,
rather than glucose, as an energy source after exercise.
Simply put, arginine makes glycogen replenishment more
efficient.

The results of these studies are meaningful for anyone
who exercises. In order to rebuild glycogen stores, maximum insulin stimulation is essential right after exercise.
The addition of protein in the correct ratio with carbohydrate, and along with arginine, can improve performance
by enhancing the insulin response, thereby promoting a
faster recovery. This is illustrated in Figure 7.1.

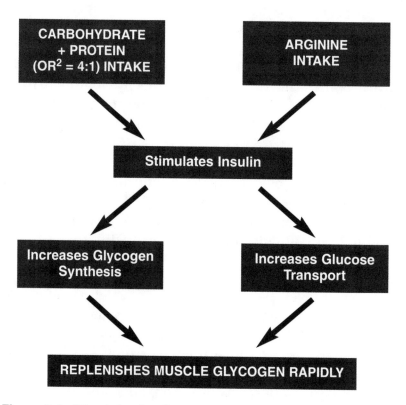

Figure 7.1. Stimulating insulin to rapidly replenish muscle glycogen

Assuming that you work out once a day for about two hours, you have approximately twenty-two "free" hours during which your body can replenish your muscle glycogen stores. Stimulating insulin without disturbing your body's other biological processes requires careful attention to your nutrient intake and balance. It must be noted that a high carbohydrate intake, above a threshold of 5 grams for every pound of body weight, will not accelerate the rate of glycogen manufactured following exercise. An ideal diet to replace glycogen and levels of essential nutrients involves moderate consumption of carbohydrate and protein. Fat intake should be minimized in the first two hours after exercise because fat, like protein, stimulates CCK, which has a negative effect on gastric emptying.

TAKING STEPS TO REPLENISH GLYCOGEN

Completely replenishing glycogen requires careful attention to your nutritional intake in the hours following exercise. Because your body responds to nutrients in different ways after exercise, it's important to balance carbohydrate, protein, and fat in the right proportions. And, as you will see, *when* you eat is just as important as *what* you eat.

The First Two Hours After Exercise

It's important to note that the type of carbohydrate you consume plays a key role in stimulating insulin response. Some foods and drinks will cause a rapid rise in your blood sugar level, allowing you to take better advantage of the increased period of insulin sensitivity during the first two hours after training or competition. You should select your post-exercise carbohydrate according to its *glycemic index,* which is an indicator of how quickly your blood sugar will rise after consumption. (See the inset "The Glycemic Index" on page 70.)

The Glycemic Index

*The **glycemic index** is a measure of the effect of carbohydrate on blood glucose levels. It compares the rise in blood sugar after a certain food is ingested with the rise in blood sugar after an equivalent amount of pure glucose, with a 100-percent glycemic index, is ingested. When you eat any food with a high glycemic index, you will experience a rapid rise in your blood sugar level, which causes your pancreas to secrete a greater amount of insulin. This is beneficial during recovery, because high-glycemic-index foods replenish glycogen more rapidly than low-glycemic-index foods. The table on page 71 categorizes some common foods according to their glycemic indexes when compared with pure glucose.*

The glycemic index is important because it indicates the effects that different foods will have on blood sugar levels. Many simple sugars, as well as breads and cereals, have high glycemic indexes. These foods replenish muscle glycogen stores rapidly because they cause an immediate rise in blood glucose, which stimulates insulin to speed glycogen synthesis and storage.

During and after workouts and competition, it's better to eat foods that cause a rapid rise in blood glucose, and an immediate insulin response, because they supply quick energy to working and recovering muscles. Other foods, such as fructose, dairy products, and some beans, have low glycemic indexes. You would probably not want to choose these foods immediately following exercise, because your blood sugar level will not rise as rapidly, making the conversion of glucose to glycogen less efficient.

Glycemic Indexes of Common Foods

High (greater than 85)	Medium (60-85)	Low (less than 60)
Bagels	Baked beans	Apples
Baked potatoes	Bananas	Applesauce
Bread, white and whole wheat	Bran cereals	Cherries
Corn syrup	Corn	Chickpeas
Cornflakes	Grapenuts	Dates
Crackers	Grapes	Figs
Glucose	Melba toast	Fructose
Honey	Oatmeal	Ice cream
Maple syrup	Orange juice	Kidney beans
Molasses	Pasta	Lentils
Raisins	Pineapple	Milk
Rice, white	Potato chips	Peaches
Rice Chex	Rye bread, whole-grain	Peanuts
Soda (sweetened with sugar)	Sucrose (white sugar)	Plums
Sports drinks (sweetened with sugar)	Watermelon	Tomato soup
	Yams	Yogurt

If you're like most people, however, you may find that exercise suppresses your appetite. Even though you're now aware of the importance of consuming carbohydrate immediately after exercise, you may be unable to eat solid foods to replenish glycogen rapidly after a workout. Fortunately, if you find that your appetite is suppressed following activity, drinks containing carbohydrate and protein, in addition to their beneficial effects on rehydration, can help you to replenish your stores of glycogen in liver and muscle tissues.

Whether you choose solid foods or liquids, your post-exercise meal or snack should be consumed as soon as possible after training or competition, in order to maximize glycogen synthesis. According to the optimum recovery ratio, about 1 gram of protein for every 4 grams of carbohydrate seems to be most effective in replenishing muscle glycogen. Try to consume 1 gram of carbohydrate for every pound of body weight, and include some protein in the proper 4 to 1 ratio. For a 150-pound athlete, this means supplementing with roughly 150 grams of carbohydrate, and about 40 grams of protein during the first two hours of post-exercise recovery. Remember to minimize fat intake because of its negative effects on gastric emptying.

Two to Four Hours After Exercise

You should consume another meal or a recovery sports drink with the optimum recovery ratio of carbohydrate to protein between two and four hours after exercise. Once again, whether the carbohydrate is in solid or liquid form does not seem to be important in terms of glycogen resynthesis. A high- to moderate-carbohydrate meal will lead to a rather rapid increase in your blood sugar level, usually within an hour. The meal should be comprised of 60 to 65 percent of calories from carbohydrate, 20 to 25 percent from fat, and about 15 percent from protein. This will increase available glycogen for exercise the next day. After this meal, however, you'll want to consume mostly low- to moderate-glycemic index foods until your pre-exercise meal the following day.

The Remaining Eighteen Hours

During the remaining eighteen hours after exercise, and before your pre-exercise meal, you should eat enough carbohydrate to equal a total intake of about 3 to 5 grams for every pound of your body weight. In other words, a 170-pound male would want to consume between 510 and 850 grams of carbohydrate during this period. A 125-pound female, on the other hand, should consume carbohydrate totaling from 375 to 625 grams. Again, the meals should include approximately 60- to 65-percent of calories from carbohydrate, 20- to 25-percent from fat, and about 15-percent from protein.

CONCLUSION

Whether you train or compete once, or several times a day, muscle and liver glycogen stores must be rebuilt quickly. The speed with which your body synthesizes glycogen determines the amount that you will ultimately be able to store. And, simply put, the more glycogen that is stored in you liver and muscles, the more energy you will have during subsequent training sessions or events. Insulin, a hormone released by the pancreas, increases the transport of glucose into your muscles, and stimulates glycogen synthesis. This enables your body to increase its energy stores at an enhanced rate.

There is a narrow window of time during which the glycogen replenishment process is most efficient. You should balance your post-exercise carbohydrate and protein according to the optimum recovery ratio, or OR^2, which is 1 gram of protein for every 4 grams of carbohydrate. This enhances the insulin response, without adversely affecting gastric emptying and rehydration.

8.

REDUCE MUSCLE AND IMMUNE-SYSTEM STRESS

"My muscles are so stiff and sore, I think I'll take today off."

Sound familiar? Most likely. For many of us, these words are all too common. Sometimes it seems as though your body rewards your endeavors to stay in top shape with sore, stiff muscles in the days following a hard workout. And, to make matters worse, you may find that even though you expect to maintain good health by exercising regularly, you are more susceptible to colds and other illness. These signs are physical evidence of the tremendous amount of stress that your muscles have undergone, resulting in muscle damage and soreness, and even reduced immunity.

Although it is not possible to completely eliminate exercise-induced muscle damage, recent research has shown that the damage due to the stress of exercise can be minimized. This research has focused on the biochemical causes of muscle stress, and has identified several key factors that can help to neutralize a number of metabolic byproducts that are culprits of muscle soreness. In addition, various studies have pinpointed specific measures that can help you to enhance your immunity, which is often weakened by exercise stress.

FREE RADICALS AND OXIDATIVE STRESS

As you learned in Chapter 4, free radicals are highly unstable molecules that can damage muscle tissue. Because the rate of oxygen consumption influences the extent of free-radical damage, also known as oxidative stress, strenuous exercise increases free-radical generation. In other words, the harder you exercise and the more oxygen you take in, the greater the generation of free radicals—and the greater the potential for muscle damage. This is, in part, the cause of your post-exercise inflammation and soreness.

Free radicals damage muscle cell membranes by attacking structural lipids (fats) known as *phospholipids*. In combination with protein, phospholipids make up all of your body's cell membranes, and the membranes of structures inside the cells, such as mitochondria. The onslaught of free radicals weakens cell membranes and affects a number of membrane-bound enzymes. In addition, the reaction of free radicals with the membrane phospholipids releases toxic substances that can inactivate other enzymes.

Free-radical damage during exercise is not an issue to be taken lightly. Prolonged endurance exercise can result in elevated muscle and whole-body levels of free radicals and the products of their reactions. Fortunately, antioxidants are your body's powerful defense against these molecular bandits.

MINIMIZING OXIDATIVE STRESS
WITH ANTIOXIDANTS

Antioxidants help to protect your body from the formation of free radicals. By neutralizing free radicals, antioxidants detoxify and protect your body against oxidative stress.

Your body produces some antioxidants as a matter of course. For example, *glutathione* is a protein produced by the liver from several amino acids. This potent antioxidant inhibits the formation of free radicals by neutralizing oxygen molecules before they can harm cells. And *superoxide dismutase* (SOD) is an enzyme that neutralizes the most common free radical, *superoxide,* and aids in the body's utilization of other antioxidants.

Your body does not produce some antioxidants, such as vitamins and minerals, so they have to be obtained from the diet. Unfortunately, even if you eat a balanced diet, it's often difficult to get enough of the antioxidants you need to counteract the effects of free radicals, particularly during periods of high stress or exercise. These circumstances may require you to supplement with extra antioxidants, such as vitamins A, C, and E, beta-carotene, and selenium. Two of these, vitamins C and E, are especially important for athletes.

Vitamin C

Recent research has shown that supplementing with vitamin C can help athletes reduce free-radical generation following exercise to prevent muscle and immune-system damage. It also aids in the production of antistress hormones, and is required for tissue growth and repair. Obviously, all of these benefits are of great importance to athletes.

One interesting study compared post-exercise muscle soreness in two groups of subjects. The experimental group was administered 3 grams of vitamin C each for three days, while none of the subjects in the control group supplemented. After the three days, both groups engaged in heavy calf exercise. The results of the study showed that subjects who had supplemented with vitamin C experienced less muscle soreness in the four days following exercise than subjects who did not take vitamin C.

In another study, subjects took either one gram per day of vitamin C or a placebo. Then, each subject completed a thirty-minute exercise session on the treadmill at 80 percent of maximum capacity. The test was repeated fourteen days later. On both the first day and the fourteenth day there was a significant reduction in free-radical formation in the group taking vitamin C when compared with the group taking the placebo.

These studies make a powerful case for the importance of incorporating vitamin C supplementation into any training program. Many researchers now recommend anywhere from 250 to 2,500 milligrams per day to neutralize free radicals and to prevent or minimize cell and muscle damage.

Vitamin E

Vitamin E functions to improve circulation, relax leg cramps, and promote tissue repair—all of which are necessary for maximum athletic performance. As an antioxidant, it prevents damage to cell membranes by inhibiting the oxidation of phospholipids. This effectively prevents the cells' protective coatings from being damaged by the assault of free radicals. Vitamin E also enhances oxygen utilization by your body, and protects other vitamins from destruction by oxygen. One study involving a treadmill test showed that supplementation with as little as 400 IU (International Units) per day decreased muscle damage by over 25 percent after exercise.

According to a recent report, vitamin E may be beneficial in preventing muscle soreness in people unaccustomed to vigorous exercise. William J. Evans, Ph.D., stated that vitamin E greatly improves the body's response to muscle injury. Evans found that 400 IU of supplemental vitamin E improved the healing process by increasing the mobilization of immune cells to damaged muscle cells, and reducing the production of oxygen free radicals. While Evans' study focused on older, active people, he concluded that younger, occasional exercisers could also benefit from antioxidant supplementation.

Conclusive evidence of vitamin E's role as a muscle protector was also collected in a study performed at Penn State University in University Park. In this instance, twelve weight-trained men were divided into two groups, with the experimental group receiving 1,200 IU of vitamin E each day, while the control group was administered a placebo pill. After two weeks, the test subjects completed a regimen of leg presses, rows, biceps curls, and squats.

The results showed that blood levels of creatine phosphokinase (CPK), an indicator of mechanical muscle damage, increased significantly in both groups in the twenty-four and forty-eight hours after exercise. At twenty-four hours, however, the increase of CPK in the group receiving vitamin E was less than that experienced by the group receiving the placebo. This means that the degree of injury caused by strenuous exercise was markedly less in those men taking vitamin E.

Laboratory research has demonstrated that vitamin E can protect against loss of muscle mass, as well. Researchers found that rats whose limbs were immobilized lost less muscle mass when they were given vitamin E as a supplement. This is akin to a person wearing an arm or leg cast, and taking vitamin E to prevent excess loss of muscle. While a certain measure of loss is inevitable when muscle use is inhibited, vitamin E clearly prevents some of the potential damage.

So what is the best dose for athletes of this powerful muscle protector? Based on the studies above, supplementation as high as 1,200 IU of vitamin E per day may be warranted to prevent muscle damage, although scientists have not yet determined the optimal intake.

The Dynamic Duo

New evidence suggests that vitamin C works synergysti-
cally with vitamin E. This means that they have a greater
impact when they work together than when they work
separately. In addition to its multitude of other functions,
vitamin C has been proven to protect antioxidants such as
vitamin E. While vitamin E scavenges for dangerous free
radicals in cell membranes, vitamin C attacks free radicals
in the body. In this way, these vitamins reinforce and
extend each other's antioxidant activity.

EXERCISE STRESS AND THE IMMUNE SYSTEM

Your immune system is responsible for identifying foreign
and potentially harmful microorganisms that have entered
your body, and then neutralizing or destroying them.
These invaders include viruses, bacteria, and fungi. White
blood cells, produced by the immune system, are your
body's first line of defense in the fight against intruders.

The stress of exercise affects your immune system by
reducing the effectiveness of white blood cells and other
immune cells. Exercise also depletes your body's supply of
the important nutrients that function to keep your body
healthy. The result is impaired healing ability, and lowered
defense against infection, both of which contribute to
decreased ability to perform during training and competition. The situation is not hopeless, however. Evidence
shows that supplementing with natural products such as
glutamine and ciwujia can keep your immune system
healthy. And exciting new studies have proven that, in
addition to providing energy for exercise, carbohydrate
drinks can help keep your immune system in top shape.

Glutamine: The Immune-System Builder

The amino acid *glutamine* functions as a source of energy

for white blood cells and other immune cells. Low levels, therefore, may weaken the immune cells, which reduces resistance to infection. In addition, glutamine plays a vital role in helping to maintain the gastrointestinal system. Although glutamine is normally manufactured in the lungs and brain, both muscle and liver cells also have this capacity. This is important because your muscles store about 60 percent of this amino acid.

In times of stress, including the physical stress of exercise, glutamine concentration in your muscles and blood plasma decreases dramatically. This is partly because physical stress causes an increase in the production of white blood cells, and more of these immune cells require more energy. At the same time, the cells of the small intestine show increased demands. These requirements cause a corresponding decrease in your blood glutamine levels. Eventually, your body's demand exceeds its capacity to produce glutamine, and it must be obtained from the diet in order to ensure healthy functioning of the immune and gastrointestinal systems. Because the glutamine produced by your body must occasionally be supplemented with dietary protein, it is considered to be a *conditionally essential* amino acid. Be aware that, although glutamine occurs naturally in a wide variety of foods, it is easily destroyed by cooking. Spinach and parsley, when eaten raw, are known to be good sources. Many sports drinks also contain supplemental glutamine.

Research with athletes has shown that endurance exercise significantly lowers blood levels of glutamine, which suggests that muscles cannot provide enough glutamine. Blood samples taken from athletes after high-intensity training sessions (between 90 and 120 percent of maximum capacity) revealed transient—but significant—decreases in blood glutamine concentrations. The same study has also reported that after only five days of a ten-day period of

Tips From the Experts

If you find that you suffer from frequent colds and other ill-nesses during training periods, don't despair! Scientists and nutritionists recommend the following measures to help boost immunity during and after exercise, and to reduce the incidence of colds and flu:

- *Eat a balanced diet to ensure healthy levels of vitamins and minerals in your body. (For recommended vitamin and mineral intakes, see Chapter 12.) Vitamin C, in par-ticular, has been shown to reduce the impact of free radi-cals on immunity when taken for several days before long events or training sessions.*

- *Make sure that you get enough sleep, especially when you engage in several days of hard training. Lack of sleep has been linked to immune system suppression.*

- *Avoid overtraining. Remember that the key to peak per-formance is to train smarter, not harder. Pushing yourself beyond your limits can have a negative impact on your ability to exercise.*

hard training, glutamine concentrations were significantly reduced, even when the athletes were at rest.

Eric Newsholme, Ph.D., and his coworkers at Oxford University were the first to point out the correlation be-tween strenuous exercise and amino-acid imbalances. A strict, strenuous training regimen that does not allow enough time for recovery may cause an athlete to suffer from over-training syndrome (OTS), which we discussed earlier in Chapter 4. As you know, this syndrome is characterized by decreased performance, depressed mood, and increased incidence of infections. OTS has been diagnosed in run-

- *Try to lower other stresses in your life. Mental and emotional stress from work and family matters and other stresses have been linked to suppressed immune function and increased risk of respiratory-tract infections.*

- *Avoid rapid weight losses during periods of hard training, because losing too much weight in too short a period of time can have a negative impact on your immune health.*

- *While training hard or tapering off exercise for an important event, it is prudent to limit your exposure to individuals who are ill. Research has also shown that heavy training is linked to suppression of **neutrophils,** the white blood cells that are part of your body's first line of defense against infections.*

  In addition to the guidelines above, you may want to consider getting a flu shot if you plan to train or compete during the winter months. Be sure to consult your physician to see if a shot is your best bet for staying flu-free during the winter months.

ners, cyclists, swimmers, skiers, and rowers, among others.

There is promising evidence, however, that glutamine supplementation may lessen the effects of overtraining. Dr. Newsholme's report suggests that overtrained athletes may, in fact, suffer from chronically low plasma glutamine concentrations. This evidence is supported further by a recent placebo-controlled study, in which athletes took 5 grams of glutamine in the first two hours after a marathon. These athletes showed a 32-percent reduction in infection rate during the seven days following competition.

Most manufacturers of sports nutrition products are

now aware of glutamine's benefits, and it has become fashionable to use it as a supplement in everything from protein powders to meal replacements. The unfortunate problem is that glutamine is expensive, so many of these "enhanced" products actually contain minimal amounts. Some manufacturers would like you to believe that a few hundred milligrams each day is adequate to maintain optimal concentrations of glutamine. In order to be effective, however, the suggested dosage falls between 8 and 20 grams daily, depending on your dietary intake, health, and how frequently and intensely you exercise. Supplementation ranging from 2 to 6 grams, two to four times per day should be enough to have a positive effect. Larger doses will most likely create an excess of glutamine, which is excreted in the urine.

Ciwujia: The Immune-System Enhancer

Ciwujia has been used in traditional Chinese medicine for almost 1,700 years to treat fatigue and boost the immune system. In the U.S., ciwujia is commonly known as Siberian ginseng (*Eleurtherococcus senticosus*), although it is not true ginseng. This root first came to the attention of researchers through published reports on its use by mountain climbers to improve work performance at high altitudes and in low-oxygen conditions.

Ciwujia has two important effects that make it a valuable supplement for muscle recovery. First, it has been shown to stimulate the immune system. This effect has been demonstrated in a number of trials in which subjects who were given ciwujia had a lower incidence of colds over a winter season. Second, it positively affects the cardiovascular system by reducing heart rate during exercise. A reduction in heart rate at the same work load level means that ciwujia reduces muscle stress.

Results from research conducted independently by

the Academy of Preventative Medicine in Beijing, China under the direction of T. Colin Campbell, Ph.D., and the Department of Physiology at the University of North Texas Health Science Center have shown that ciwujia can also improve workout performance through a carbohydrate-sparing action. In one trial, eight healthy male adults underwent aerobic and anaerobic assessments on a stationary bicycle. Following supplementation with ciwujia, subjects showed a decrease in lactic acid levels ranging from 31 to 33 percent—a decrease that became more pronounced at higher energy workloads. This occurred because subjects utilized other fuels, such as fat, instead of carbohydrate.

Over the course of the study, the average increase in the use of fat for energy in the group taking ciwujia was slightly more than 43 percent. These results indicate that ciwujia offers significant benefits during exercise. By shifting the energy source from carbohydrate to fat during exercise, ciwujia increases fat metabolism, which spares glycogen and delays lactic-acid buildup. Therefore, ciwujia appears to have a place in the nutrition program of any athlete who wants to optimize his or her metabolism during exercise, and to reduce exercise-induced immune stress.

Carbohydrate: The Immune-System Crusader

It's safe to say that almost every athlete knows about the energy boost that carbohydrate can provide, before and during exercise. But encouraging new studies have shown that carbohydrate can also help the body to combat the stress of hard training, which can suppress immune system function for several hours following a workout. Recent research by Dr. David Nieman and his coworkers from Appalachian State University in North Carolina has shown that athletes can lower immune stress by drinking a carbohydrate-containing sports drink. These results were achieved in subjects who consumed 8 ounces of the drink every fifteen minutes during exercise lasting several hours.

Certain types of white blood cells associated with immune stress are increased in response to endurance exercise. Dr. Nieman found that this increase was reduced when the subjects drank a sports drink as opposed to an artificially flavored placebo drink, containing no active ingredients.

The same research team has also investigated the body's release of cortisol in response to the stress of exercise. Dr. Nieman's research found that cortisol levels were lower after exercise when the subjects consumed a sports drink containing carbohydrate during activity. Therefore, carbohydrate supplementation is believed to blunt the rise of cortisol in response to stress. Cortisol, as you remember, increases protein use during long-term exercise, which weakens muscles.

"Our research shows that sports drinks not only provide carbohydrate energy during exercise, but supports the link between sports drinks and less stress to the immune system," says Dr. Nieman. "Carbohydrate drinks of about 6-percent to 10-percent carbohydrate [per 100 milliliters of water] consumed during exercise will not eliminate the stress of training, but our research and the work of others show they can reduce the increase of several byproducts of stress and hard exercise." Therefore, carbohydrate can be a good addition to your anti-stress arsenal. Figure 8.1 on page 87 provides a brief summary on the principles of reducing muscle and immune-system stress.

CONCLUSION

Many experts now recommend that you enhance your body's natural antioxidants, as well as your immune system, with vitamin, mineral, herb, and amino acid supplements. Available research data has made it abundantly clear that these supplements are extremely important to

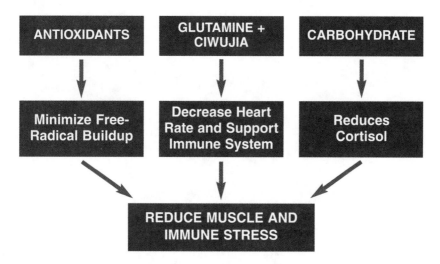

Figure 8.1. The key factors in reducing muscle and immune-system stress

protect your muscles and maintain overall health—and that most athletes are probably not getting enough. Given the evidence concerning the harmful effects of free radicals, and immune system suppression due to training, your best offense is a healthy, balanced diet, supplemented with a solid vitamin, mineral, and herbal defense. And don't underestimate the benefits of supplementing with a recovery drink containing carbohydrate, glutamine, and antioxidants after hard training to neutralize free radicals and give your immune system a boost.

9.

REBUILD MUSCLE PROTEIN

Through the years, protein has undoubtedly been one of the most widely discussed nutrients in the sports world. Some might say that it is also one of the most misunderstood nutrients. Bodybuilders believe they can never get enough of it, endurance athletes generally don't get enough of it, and nutritionists will be the first to tell you that the average American diet contains far too much protein, in proportion to other nutrients. In the face of so many conflicting viewpoints, how do you know if you're getting enough protein to improve your strength and performance—or even enough to maintain your overall health?

Fortunately, there are a few facts that we can all agree upon. As we discussed in Chapter 2, protein is a nutrient with various and diverse functions in the body. It is required for the growth, maintenance, and repair of all cells, and for the production of enzymes and hormones. And because protein is an essential component of muscle structure, sufficient amounts are required for recovery after exercise, to ensure proper repair and development of your muscle cells.

PROTEIN AS A FUEL SOURCE

The body tends to spare protein as a fuel source because of the nutrient's numerous structural and metabolic functions. However, when glycogen stores run low, some amino acids from muscle tissue are used for energy, even though the body can depend, in part, on the fat that it has stored. This generally occurs during intensive exercise, such as powerlifting or endurance activities. Because protein is a component of muscle tissue, which is functional, this breakdown of muscle tissue has a negative impact on muscle strength and endurance.

As you learned in Chapter 4, your adrenal glands secrete the hormone cortisol in response to physical stress such as exercise. Cortisol extracts protein from muscle tissues in order to help mobilize energy for your body. As exercise duration increases, more protein is robbed from your muscles to meet your body's demand for energy, which, in turn, increases the need for protein consumption after exercise. By stimulating insulin with carbohydrate supplementation during exercise and recovery, the cortisol response to muscle stress is blunted.

Branched-Chain Amino Acids

During hard exercise bouts, your body uses certain amino acids for fuel. The muscles use the branched-chain amino acids (BCAAs) isoleucine, leucine, and valine to supply a limited amount of energy during strenuous exercise.

Together, BCAAs make up a significant part of your body's muscle protein. In addition to providing some fuel for exercise, they are involved in energy production during exercise, and they promote the manufacture and growth of muscle tissue. Therefore, they are important components of the R^4 System.

For many years, researchers believed that all three BCAAs were used in equal proportions to provide energy. However, it has recently been discovered that leucine is used in far greater amounts during exercise and rest alike. Leucine is thought to stimulate the release of insulin, thereby increasing protein synthesis during activity and recovery.

Researchers have still not determined if it is necessary to supplement with large quantities of branched-chain amino acids. At this time, it does not seem that there is a real need to supplement with any of the BCAAs in excess of those amounts provided by a quality carbohydrate and protein supplement.

DO YOU NEED MORE PROTEIN?

Many athletes are able to obtain adequate amounts of protein by eating a healthy, balanced diet. Athletes who engage in sports that depend more heavily on protein for energy, however, may need to increase their protein intake, or use supplements to compensate for what their diets cannot provide. Some activities that require a greater quantity of protein for energy are listed below.

❑ **Endurance sports:** Athletes who regularly push themselves to their absolute physical limits, such as distance runners, triathletes, and competitive cyclists, can seriously tax their carbohydrate fuel reserves. As these carbohydrate stores diminish, more and more protein is burned as an alternative fuel source. Up to 10 percent of an athlete's energy supply during prolonged exercise may, in fact, come from protein sources. In addition to this, protein is necessary to repair tissues damaged by the wear and tear of the exercise itself.

❑ **Heavy physical training:** Athletes working hard in any sport for ninety minutes or more on a daily basis will also burn protein as fuel, causing them to experience the same wear-and-tear damage to muscle tissue as endurance athletes. Extra protein can help to offset tissue damage due to exercise, and can provide a needed boost to rebuild muscle protein.

❏ **Heavy weight training:** Athletes who engage in strenuous weightlifting need protein to repair muscle tissue that is catabolized during training. Extra protein also helps muscles to adapt to the progressive physical stress that is a natural element in training with weights. A weightlifter's body adapts to increasing stress by synthesizing more protein in each muscle cell, in order to build stronger muscles that can handle more stress. A greater proportion of protein in muscle tissues translates into stronger muscle contractions. Therefore, the athlete will be able to lift the same weight with greater ease during subsequent workouts.

❏ **Sports requiring calorie-restricted diets:** Wrestlers, dancers, jockeys, boxers, and others who have to deal with weigh-ins and weight classes often subject themselves to low-calorie diets for long periods of time. Unable to consume a healthy balance of nutrients, these athletes run short of glycogen stores in less time than athletes who consume sufficient nutrients to maintain their energy levels, and burn higher quantities of protein as fuel during training and performance. These athletes need more protein in their diets to replenish muscle protein that is burned as fuel, as well as to rebuild muscle tissue that is damaged during exercise.

Untrained muscles, or muscles that are unused to a specific activity or level of intensity, are more susceptible to damage. Therefore, athletes just beginning an exercise program, as well as athletes expanding significantly on their current program, are especially in need of extra protein. But be aware that any athlete who is trying to ensure adequate protein intake needs to eat just the right amount to minimize the formation of metabolic waste products. When too much protein is consumed, the body converts the excess to fat and increases the blood levels of ammonia and uric acid. Ammonia and uric acid are toxic metabolic waste products. The athlete's goal, therefore, is to maintain proper, balanced protein intake.

ENHANCING PROTEIN SYNTHESIS

The breakdown of protein for energy is a setback for athletes who have been training hard to make gains. When muscle glycogen depletion causes the body to use amino acids as a source of energy, it cannot also use these amino acids for building and maintaining muscle mass and strength. The result is a slower rate of muscle development, or even decreased performance capacity. In such cases, carbohydrate and protein supplementation may be just the formula to rebuild muscle protein. A summary of this principle is presented in Figure 9.1 on page 94.

Insulin: The Jack of All Trades

Insulin is an essential factor in maintaining a healthy protein balance. It increases protein synthesis by facilitating the transport of amino acids into muscle cells, where they can be used to synthesize proteins for structural purposes. Research has clearly demonstrated the advantages of taking a carbohydrate-protein supplement after exercise in order to increase protein synthesis. These supplements help your body to sustain an environment conducive to muscle growth and development, which carbohydrate supplementation alone cannot provide.

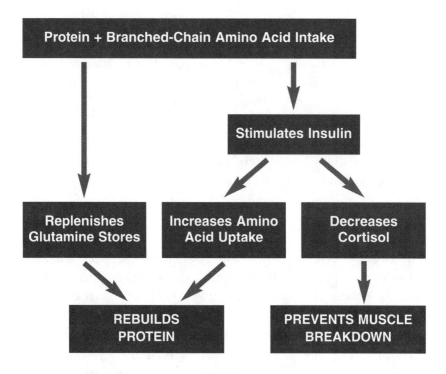

Figure 9.1. Rebuilding muscle tissues with protein and amino acid supplementation

Glutamine: It's Not Just for Immunity, Anymore

When we first discussed glutamine in Chapter 8, it was in terms of its role in maintaining healthy immune function. But since the majority of this amino acid is made in the muscles, it is also readily available when needed for the synthesis of skeletal muscle proteins. However, during times of stress, such as the physical stress of exercise, as much as one-third of the glutamine present in the muscles may be released to meet the needs of the immune system, leading to the loss of skeletal muscle.

Supplementing with glutamine is known to produce a strong anticatabolic effect, which counteracts some of the muscle breakdown that accompanies strenuous exercise.

High glutamine levels in muscle cells stimulate the entry of other amino acids into the cells. Thus, glutamine is considered to be an anabolic, or constructive, amino acid. In the scientific community there is a growing interest in glutamine because of its activity in preserving muscle mass.

CONCLUSION

During strenuous or long-term exercise, protein—which is mainly a structural and functional nutrient in the body—is called upon to provide fuel for activity. This can have a detrimental effect for two reasons. First, amino acids that would otherwise be used to build and repair muscle tissues are instead used for energy production. Second, the physical stress of exercise stimulates the release of the body's stress hormone, cortisol, which breaks down structural protein so that it can be mobilized for energy. This results in a decrease in strength, because some amount of muscle mass is lost.

Immediately following exercise, a rebuilding process is initiated to repair muscle proteins damaged during exercise. Recent evidence suggests that insulin is a strong stimulus for the muscle rebuilding process because it increases amino acid transport into muscles. By blunting the rise of cortisol, insulin also minimizes protein breakdown from the muscles. In addition to this, glutamine is an anabolic amino acid that can counteract some of the muscle loss due to exercise.

10.

MAKING SCIENCE PRACTICAL: THE R^4 SYSTEM DRINK

B y now it should be quite clear to you that training isn't only about exercise. Recovery is just as important for performance. Why? Because the degree to which you restore your body's fluid balance, replenish energy, minimize muscle stress, and rebuild protein determines the level at which you'll perform the next day.

According to Dave Scott, six-time winner of the Ironman Triathlon, smart athletes take steps to optimize recovery by consuming the right nutrients at the right times, during and after exercise. If you guide your body's recovery with proper nutrition, he says, "you'll be a lot more consistent in your training, and you'll arrive at a higher level in your performance."

The R^4 System represents an innovation in sports nutrition. What makes this model so revolutionary is that it goes beyond rehydration and carbohydrate loading to provide a comprehensive nutritional plan for recovery. The R^4 System is based on significant studies conducted over the last decade, which have shown that:

- Insulin is the master recovery hormone that, when stimulated, can rapidly replenish muscle glycogen and re-build muscle protein.

- Protein and specific amino acids, such as branched-chain amino acids and arginine, can maximally stimulate insulin when consumed in the correct ratio with carbohydrate.

- Antioxidants can minimize soreness and speed recovery by reducing free-radical damage, also known as oxidative stress.

- Amino acids and certain natural supplements can help reduce muscle and immune-system stress during and after exercise.

By maximizing recovery with the principles detailed in the previous chapters, you'll find that it's possible to make great strides in reaching your performance goals.

Now that we have a better understanding of muscle recovery, the challenge is to formulate practical products that incorporate the principles of the R^4 System for athletes of all levels and experience. The sports nutrition market is glutted with products guaranteed to help you extend your endurance and increase your level of performance. But is the product you're using based on the revolutionary ideas above, or is it formulated according to twenty-year-old science? This chapter will open your eyes to what you *should* be looking for in a sports drink.

THE SPORTS DRINK REVOLUTION

When it comes to sports drinks, many manufacturers are only partly aware of what a product must contain in order to be truly effective. Carbohydrate and electrolytes have been much touted as the most essential ingredients in any sports drink. However, although ingredients such as carbohydrate are certainly essential, numerous manufacturers have adopted the philosophy that more is better—which is not necessarily the case. For example, simply adding more carbohydrate without stimulating insulin may not be effective in rapidly replenishing glycogen stores, because insulin is a critical factor in transporting glucose to muscles for glycogen synthesis. And while protein is another fundamental component, some manufacturers include large amounts, exceeding the optimum recovery ratio. Others do not include any protein. As we saw in Chapter 7, some of these factors can have a negative impact on gastric emptying, which impedes hydration and electrolyte replenishment during and after exercise.

During exercise, you need a concentrated source of nutrient fuel that your body can digest rapidly, to give you quick energy for that burst off the line, or sprint to the ball. And you also need adequate fuel to keep you going for hours at a time. Carbohydrate and electrolytes alone are not enough to ensure adequate support of muscle metabolism during exercise to delay fatigue, or to prevent oxidative stress. And during recovery, you need a product that will enhance glycogen synthesis to replenish energy stores, provide protein to rebuild and repair muscles, and protect your immune system.

In 1997, I participated in a conference with six leading exercise physiologists to brainstorm about what factors could lead to an improved and cutting-edge sports drink. We reasoned that a product based on the latest science would offer major advantages over available sports nutrition products because it would combine all of the benefits of the R⁴ System in one convenient source. In addition to providing the benefits of rehydration and enhanced energy, the drink would be specially formulated to significantly improve performance by enhancing the insulin response to speed muscle glycogen replenishment; protecting muscles cells from free-radical damage, thereby reducing muscle soreness; and rebuilding damaged muscle tissues with protein and amino acid supplementation. The next step was to see how the R^4 System Drink would fare in field tests. The formulation which was tested is shown in Figure 10.1.

WEIGHING THE EVIDENCE

The first trial was conducted by Dr. Peter Raven, a Professor of Physiology at the University of North Texas State, and Dr. John Ivy, a Professor of Physiology at the University of Texas at Austin. In this study, subjects were depleted of muscle glycogen through exercise, and

	Restore Electrolytes	Replenish Glycogen	Reduce Muscle Stress	Rebuild Muscle Protein
Potassium	●			
Sodium	●			
Magnesium	●			
High Glycemic Carbohydrate		●		
Carbohydrate/Protein (OR^2 = 4:1)		●		
Arginine		●		
Vitamin E			●	
Vitamin C			●	
Ciwujia			●	
Glutamine			●	●
Branched-Chain Amino Acids				●
Whey Protein				●

Figure 10.1. The R^4 System Drink Formula

then were provided either the R^4 System Drink or a leading sports drink during recovery. Following the recovery
phase, subjects underwent a performance bout measuring
how long they could exercise at 85 percent of maximum
capacity.

I conducted the second trial in collaboration with Dr.
John Seifert, Professor of Physiology at St. Cloud State
University. For this test, ten well-trained athletes completed a simulated duathalon. In the first phase, subjects ran
on a treadmill at moderate intensity (75 percent of their
maximum capacity) for forty-five minutes. The second
phase was a ten-minute rest period, during which the subjects consumed either the R^4 System Drink or the leading
sports drink. Then, in the third phase, the subjects cycled
for thirty minutes at 75 percent of their maximum capacity.
At the end of the cycling phase, all subjects underwent a
time trial in which they completed a given amount of
cycling work in as short a time as they could.

The researchers found that the R^4 System Drink, when
compared with the leading sports drink:

❑ **Increased endurance performance up to 55 percent.**
This is the most important aspect of the R^4 System. By
accelerating the recovery process through rapid replenishment of glycogen stores, the R^4 System Drink significantly improved muscle performance. The subjects
were not only able to exercise longer, but they also felt
less fatigue, as evidenced by the fact that the ratings of
perceived exertion were lower.

❑ **Reduced the total buildup of free radicals by 69 percent.** The latest studies have shown that free radical
build-up is one of the causes of post-exercise muscle
damage and soreness.

❑ **Reduced muscle damage by 36 percent.** As you will
recall, creatine phosphokinase (CPK) is a marker of

post-exercise muscle damage. CPK levels in the R^4 group were almost 40 percent lower in the twenty-four hours after exercise, when compared with the group that consumed the leading sports drink.

❏ **Stimulated average insulin levels by 70 percent.** Insulin stimulation is an important cornerstone of the R^4 System because of its importance in the post-recovery process. By stimulating insulin, the R^4 System Drink speeds the replenishment of glycogen stores. Based on recent studies, the drink appears to offer a benefit in blunting the rise in cortisol levels and repairing proteins damaged during exericse.

❏ **Decreased average heart rate.** By lowering heart rate, the R^4 System Drink decreases stress on the cardiovascular system.

❏ **Produced equivalent rates of rehydration.** Although protein, in combination with carbohydrate, has been proven to stimulate insulin, it can also slow gastric emptying. This is why the ratio of protein to carbohydrate is so important. The R^4 System Drink contains the optimum recovery ratio (OR^2) of 4 grams of carbohydrate to 1 gram of protein. This ratio provides the muscle cells with the benefits of protein without hindering the rehydration process.

One last point that applies to all sports drinks: it has to taste good if consumers are going to drink it. Participants in these trials rated the R^4 System Drink statistically equal in taste to the leading sports drink product.

CONCLUSION

The most up-to-date research has proven that sports drinks formulated to optimize recovery can help athletes increase

Selecting a Sports Drink

When you select a sports drink for optimal recovery, you should be certain that you get what you pay for. That's not so easy when you find yourself standing before a bounty of energy and recovery drinks, each one with its own remarkable claim. To help you narrow down your options, you can evaluate possible contenders according to the following criteria:

- *Does the drink contain adequate amounts of antioxidants to be effective? Vitamins C and E, especially, have been research-proven to reduce oxidative stress and free-radical damage during and after exercise.*

- *Does the drink contain carbohydrate and protein in the optimal recovery ratio of 4 grams of carbohydrate to 1 gram of protein? Are these ingredients included in the proper amounts to maximize post-exercise insulin levels?*

- *Does the drink contain natural herbs and the amino acid glutamine to help minimize immune-system stress?*

- *Does the drink contain adequate levels of the electrolytes sodium, chloride, potassium, and magnesium? (Refer to the chart on page 62.)*

An educated consumer is most likely to choose a product that suits his or her needs. Be certain to check the nutrition labels and ingredient lists for each product that you consider buying. This will help you to make sure the product you select meets the criteria above for what constitutes an effective sports drink for optimal recovery.

muscle gains and improve performance. Few products are available, however, that can truly claim to maximize recovery. While many provide adequate ingredients for rehydration, and nutrition for energy *during* exercise, they do not enhance recovery *after* exercise.

In order for any drink to be effective, it has to stimulate insulin to rapidly replenish glycogen stores and rebuild muscle protein. In addition, a drink that is formulated according to recent studies will contain antioxidants to combat free-radical damage and, as a result, minimize muscle soreness. An ideal drink, in short, should maximize recovery according to the principles of the R^4 System, in order to minimize muscle fatigue and muscle damage.

PART III

GOING THE EXTRA MILE

Optimal muscle recovery is fundamental to achieving athletic success. By putting the principles of the R^4 System into practice, you'll be able to replenish energy stores, minimize muscle soreness, and protect your immune system so that you can perform at peak capacity every time you exercise. However, there are measures that you can take, above and beyond the guidelines presented by the R^4 System, that can be equally important in helping you to reach—or even exceed—your performance goals.

Part III will show you how to go the extra mile to ensure peak performance when you train or compete. It begins with a complete guide to eating a healthy, balanced diet to maintain overall good health. This is followed by a look at some performance-enhancing supplements that can help your body to produce more energy, and to build and repair muscles. You will also learn about effective methods of carbohydrate loading prior to competition to delay physical fatigue during your event. And, in the last chapter, you'll find an in-depth discussion on massage, stretching, and other nonnutritional methods for restoring your muscles to health, and for maintaining muscle strength and flexibility.

11.

NUTRITION FOR
EVERY DAY

Nutrition for performance is not just about what you eat directly before or after exercise to help you run faster, cycle harder, or extend your training session. Every day, you have to eat a selection of foods that supplies essential nutrients and energy just to carry out your day-to-day activities. As an athlete, you want to optimize your daily diet so that you have additional energy for exercise, as well as the nutrients you need to aid your body's building and repair processes. This means that you have to eat more of the right foods, in specific proportions, to ensure good health and maximum performance.

There are six categories of nutrients that your body needs for survival. The four basic nutrients—also known as macronutrients—are water, carbohydrate, fat, and protein. (The two remaining classes of nutrients are vitamins and minerals, which we will discuss in the following chapter.) To ensure maximum performance, both in your everyday routine and your training program, you need to include the healthiest forms of these nutrients in your diet. In addition, it's important to maintain the proper balance of macronutrients for your sport and activity level.

The unfortunate fact is that the typical American diet includes far too high a proportion of fat, sodium, and sugar. Although this kind of diet is adequate for everyday life, it's clearly not *nutritious*—that is, it doesn't provide your body with the right nutrients in the correct amounts for optimum health. What's more, an excess of high-fat, sugar-sweetened foods can lead to numerous health problems, including heart disease, diabetes, and certain types of cancer.

This chapter focuses on the four basic nutrients that are essential for optimal health and performance, paying particular attention to the energy-yielding nutrients carbohydrate, fat, and protein. The material provides general guidelines to help you include more of the "good" forms of these nutrients in your daily diet, not only to prevent disease, but to maintain overall good health.

WATER

Of the four basic nutrients, water is the most essential in maintaining life. Although it contains no energy in the form of calories, water is involved in almost every function of the body. Therefore, replacing water that is continuously lost through sweating and excretion is very important. While the body can survive for several weeks without food, it cannot survive for more than a few days without water.

CARBOHYDRATE

Carbohydrate is the body's primary energy source for all activities. Through digestion and metabolism, carbohydrate is broken down into glucose molecules, which can be used for immediate energy, or stored as glycogen. In previous chapters we focused on stimulating insulin with carbohydrate and protein—in the proper ratio—to replenish glycogen rapidly. As you will remember, the first two hours after exercise are a period of maximum insulin sensitivity, when glycogen synthesis occurs at a faster-than-normal rate to give your body a "jump start" in replenishing glycogen. Your body continues to rebuild energy stores in the hours after, however, so it's important to optimize your carbohydrate intake during this time to ensure enough energy for school- or work-related activities and training sessions alike.

Optimizing carbohydrate intake means more than just consuming adequate amounts to replenish glycogen. Athletes also need to consider the types of carbohydrates they eat, and when they eat them. For example, simple carbohydrates consist of *monosaccharides*, which are single sugar molecules. Monosaccharides such as glucose do not need to be broken down, and therefore enter the bloodstream immediately, providing a quick supply of energy. Simple carbohydrates, when consumed just before and during exercise, can maintain blood sugar for energy and spare glycogen. On the other hand, complex carbohydrates, including starch and glycogen, are composed of long chains of glucose molecules, known as *polysaccharides*. These chains have to be broken down before your body can use the glucose, so complex carbohydrates supply your body with a steady supply of energy for a longer duration.

Fiber is a type of polysaccharide that your body cannot break down for energy. However, dietary fiber, which is also called *roughage*, helps the intestines to function efficiently, and aids absorption of sugars into the bloodstream. Fiber-rich diets also promote a feeling of satiety, or fullness. In addition, research has shown that people who eat high-fiber diets experience reduced rates of cardiovascular disease, colon cancer, and diabetes.

Dietary Guidelines for Carbohydrate

For maximum performance, you should consume about 60 percent of your total daily calories from carbohydrate, keeping in mind that carbohydrate contains 4 calories per gram. For example, if your daily requirement is 2,400 calories, you would take in 1,440 calories from carbohydrate each day. To calculate your required carbohydrate intake, simply multiply your total daily calories by 0.60, or 60 percent. You can achieve roughly the same intake by consuming 3 to 5 grams of carbohyrate for every pound of your body weight.

When you choose carbohydrate-rich foods for your diet, try to select unrefined foods such as fruits, vegetables, peas, beans, pasta, and whole-grain products. It's wise to avoid processed foods, including soft drinks, desserts, candy, and sugar, which offer few—if any—of the vitamins and minerals that are important to your health. Another problem is that foods high in refined simple sugars are often high in fat, which should be limited in a healthy diet. Be aware that it's important not to skip meals because this may lead to low blood glucose, which will in turn compromise protein and glycogen synthesis.

During my work with the National Cycling Team training camps at the Olympic Training Center in Colorado Springs, Colorado, I was surprised to find that many athletes did not know how to select high-carbohydrate foods. Often, the foods that athletes believe are high in carbohydrates are instead high in fat. Fortunately, there's an easy method for separating the high-carbohydrate foods from their imposters.

Let's assume, for example, that you choose a chocolate croissant for breakfast. It has 25 grams of carbohydrate and 260 calories per serving (serving size is one croissant). You can calculate the percentage of carbohydrate in the croissant in two simple steps:

1. First, multiply the number of grams of carbohydrate per serving by four:

$$25 \times 4 = 100$$

This gives you the total number of carbohydrate calories per serving.

2. Now, divide the number of carbohydrate calories by the total number of calories per serving:

$$100 \div 260 = .38 \text{ or } 38 \text{ percent}$$

As you can see above, your chocolate croissant is 38-percent carbohydrate. Clearly, this is *not* a high-carbohydrate food.

FAT

Lately, there has been a great deal of confusion concerning the place that fats have in the diet. Reports linking high-fat diets to illnesses such as heart disease, certain cancers, and diabetes have driven some people to reduce the fat in their diets to very low levels. However, studies have shown that this extreme can be unhealthy, as well. Why? The fact is that some amount of dietary fat is essential for good health. Besides being your body's most concentrated source of energy, fat provides insulation, and acts as protective padding for your bones and internal organs. And fats known as phospholipids are components of all cell membranes and other cellular structures, such as mitochondria.

A diet containing a moderate amount of fat is important for athletes who wish to maximize their performance and who need to increase their calorie consumption. Many athletes do not eat enough fat simply because they eat a high-carbohydrate diet, including greater than 70 percent of calories from carbohydrate on a regular basis. In addition, some athletes are "fat phobics"—they cut back on their intake of fat because they have been led to believe that all fat is bad for their health. So while they train long and hard in an effort to stimulate their muscles' fat utilization, they often eat a diet depleted of fat, which sends the conflicting signal to their muscles that building extra machinery for metabolizing fat is a waste of cellular energy and space.

Unfortunately, the typical American diet includes too much total fat, too much of the wrong kinds of fats, and too little of the right kinds. The solution to this dietary dilemma, then, is not to simply cut fat out of your diet. Instead, it's important to have a working knowledge about some of the different types of fats, and how they affect or are utilized by the body.

Fatty Acids

As we first discussed in Chapter 2, fats are composed of fatty acids. There are three major types of fatty acids found in the diet and in the body—saturated, polyunsaturated, and monounsaturated.

Saturated fatty acids tend to be solid at room temperature. They are found mainly in animal products, including whole milk, cream, and cheese, and fatty meats. A diet high in saturated fat increases the amount of cholesterol circulating in the blood. Therefore, including too many saturated fats in the diet can significantly raise the blood cholesterol level, especially the level of the "bad" low-density lipoprotein (LDL) cholesterol.

Polyunsaturated fatty acids are generally liquid at room temperature, and are found in corn, soybean, safflower, and sunflower oils. Although these fats have been shown to reduce total blood cholesterol level, they may also lower the level of the "good" high-density lipoprotein (HDL) cholesterol. *Monounsaturated fatty acids,* on the other hand, seem to lower LDL cholesterol without affecting HDL cholesterol. Olive, peanut, and canola oils have high amounts of monounsaturates.

Essential Fatty Acids

Essential fatty acids (EFAs) are necessary for rebuilding and producing new cells, and for maintaining proper brain and nervous-system function. Although they are essential for health, EFAs cannot be made by the body—they must be obtained from the diet. Omega-3 and omega-6 fats are the two EFAs that we require for good health. Omitting these fatty acids from the diet can result in serious health problems.

Omega-3 EFAs, in particular, have been found to reduce the risk of heart disease and to lower blood pressure. The problem is that many of us don't include enough of the omega-3s in our diets. It's not that these EFAs don't occur naturally in a variety of foods. We just don't eat enough of the foods that are good sources of omega-3s, such as fresh deepwater fish, fish oil, and certain vegetable oils, including canola, flaxseed, and walnut oils.

In contrast to omega-3 fatty acids, the omega-6 EFAs are much more available. *Omega-6* EFAs are found primarily in raw nuts, seeds, and legumes, and in unsaturated vegetable oils, such as grape seed oil, primrose oil, sesame oil, and soybean oil. They also occur in some amount in chicken, turkey, lamb, and pork. While no one knows the exact amount of omega-3 and omega-6 fats needed for optimal health, researchers are warning us to be careful to maintain a good balance of these EFAs. A healthy ratio is said to be no more than three times more omega-6 than omega-3 fatty acids. High levels of omega-6 fatty acids, out of balance with the omega-3s, can promote health problems such as heart disease, asthma, autoimmune diseases, diabetes, and weakened nerve fibers.

Dietary Guidelines for Fat

Because some amount of fat is necessary to maintain optimum health, your daily diet should include about 25 percent of calories from fat. Each gram of fat contains 9 calories, making it your body's most concentrated source of energy, with more than twice the energy of a gram of carbohydrate. To figure out your fat allowance, multiply your total calorie intake per day by 0.25, or 25 percent. Assuming, once again, that your total calorie requirement is 2,400 calories per day, you should consume 600 calories from fat for optimum health. This equals roughly 67 grams of fat daily. When calculating your daily fat intake, keep in mind that 1 teaspoon of fat equals 5 grams, which equals 45 calories; and 1 tablespoon of fat equals 15 grams, which equals 135 calories.

In general, endurance athletes need to maintain higher levels of fat intake than do power athletes. It's important to remember, however, that all athletes should focus on reducing their saturated-fat intake, and increasing their intake of the essential fatty acids, particularly the omega-3s. The following tips can help you to increase your EFA intake:

- Use olive and canola oils when cooking, instead of margarine and butter.

- Aim to eat at least 3 to 9 ounces of fish a week.

- Use walnuts, almonds, and other nuts more frequently as a topping for cereal, yogurt, and salads.

- Add ground flaxseed oil to your diet.

- Select whole-grain products over refined versions for small amounts of essential fats.

As a general rule, you should try to avoid—or at least try to lower your intake of—whole milk products, butter, egg yolks, cream cheese, and fatty meats such as bacon, hot dogs, bologna, and hamburgers. Coconut and palm oils, as well as organ meats, including kidney and liver, are also foods that you should eat only occasionally. These foods are all high in saturated fatty acids and cholesterol. Instead, eat lean meats such as fish, chicken, and turkey; egg whites; and skim-milk products.

Regarding sources of pure fat, such as oils, food sources high in polyunsaturated fats should be substituted for food sources high in saturated fats. Fat sources to avoid include butter, bacon fat, cream, mayonnaise, and mayonnaise-based salad dressings.

PROTEIN

So far, when we have discussed protein, it has been in terms of structural units called amino acids. Of the more than 20 amino acids that have been identified, nine have been identified as essential amino acids, which cannot be manufactured by the body. Essential amino acids, there-fore, must be obtained from dietary sources. *Complete proteins* are proteins that contain all of the nine essential amino acids in sufficient amounts for adequate growth and development. Meat, fish, dairy products, and eggs have complete proteins.

Incomplete proteins are missing one or more of the essential amino acids, which negatively affects growth and developmental rates. However, your body can actually manufacture complete proteins if you consume a variety of plant foods, such as beans, grains, vegetables, fruits, nuts, and seeds, as well as sufficient calories every day. This is good news for vegetarians, who do not eat animal foods to obtain complete proteins. Evidence even suggests that well-balanced vegetarian meals may decrease the risk of heart disease and cancer, because they're lower in fat and higher in complex carbohydrates than the typical Amer-ican diet.

Dietary Guidelines for Protein

You should aim to consume about 15 percent of your total calorie intake from protein. Simply multiply your daily caloric intake by 0.15, or 15 percent, to calculate your protein requirement. Therefore, if you take in 2,400 calories per day, 360 of those calories should come from protein. As with carbohydrate, protein has about 4 calories per gram.

When you calculate your protein requirement, remember to take into consideration the duration and intensity of your activity. Some types of exercise require athletes to consume more calories from protein. Athletes who exercise for several hours at a time can actually lose muscle mass because they burn a high percentage of protein for fuel. To help maintain muscle mass, these athletes may benefit from up to 1 gram of protein for every pound of body weight.

One of the challenges with protein intake is to choose protein sources that are healthy and complete. Animal foods, such as dairy products, meat, and eggs, provide all the essential amino acids that you need to build and develop muscle. However, these foods can add an unhealthy amount of the wrong kinds of fats to your diet. A diet loaded with fat is an *atherogenic diet*, meaning that it increases your risk for heart disease. Your best bet, then, is to choose lean meats, such as poultry and lean red meat from which the fat has been trimmed; low-fat dairy products, including low-fat or skim milk; and most fishes and shellfishes. Remember that including more fish in your diet will also help you to boost your intake of the essential fatty acids.

Foods derived from plants, such as fruits, vegetables, and grains are typically low in fat and cholesterol. Unfortunately, unlike animal proteins, plant proteins are generally incomplete in their essential-amino-acid content. It's possible to get an adequate balance of these amino acids, however, by combining different plant proteins. Eating fruits, vegetables, and grains in the proper combinations will enable you to get all of the amino acids you need to build muscle, without adding as much fat as animal proteins. A popular grain-and-vegetable combination is brown rice and corn. Peas and carrots are a good combination for complete proteins from legumes and vegetables. And even a peanut butter sandwich is sufficient for a grain-and-legume complete-protein combination.

Protein Supplements

In order to maintain muscle mass, athletes need to take in adequate protein to offset some of what is catabolized for energy during exercise. This is not always easy. In fact, it's not uncommon for certain types of athletes, such as endurance athletes and weighlifters, to have difficulty consuming enough protein to meet their daily requirements—and this may not be from lack of trying! For athletes who require large quantities of protein daily, including these amounts in the diet may be a challenge. In these cases, a protein supplement may be just the answer.

If you think that you need to give your dietary protein intake a supplemental boost, keep in mind that protein consumed in excess is not converted to muscle. Instead, it's often converted to fat. Therefore, you should take special care to eat just the right amount for your weight and activity level.

Carbohydrate-Protein Supplements

If you need extra protein, you may benefit from the convenience of a mixed carbohydrate-protein supplement. These products are available in all shapes, sizes, and combinations. The important thing to remember is to choose a supplement that's healthy and low in fat. A complete prod-

Investigating the 40–30–30 Diet

The 40–30–30 diet has recently become a popular nutritional regimen in the sports and fitness world. Athletes on this diet plan obtain 40 percent of their calories from carbohydrate, 30 percent from fat, and 30 percent from protein, in contrast to the 60–25–15 ratio that has traditionally been recommended by nutritionists. Supporters of the 40–30–30 plan say that decreasing carbohydrate intake and boosting protein consumption will enable dieters to burn more fat. For athletes, this translates into a glycogen-sparing effect, which can extend endurance.

The theory behind the 40–30–30 diet is that a lower carbohydrate intake, coupled with an increased percentage of protein, will help to keep insulin levels low in the blood. From what you've already learned about insulin's importance in glycogen manufacture and storage, you might be wondering what benefits low insulin levels would offer. While insulin is essential for processing carbohydrate, it has also been shown to inhibit fat metabolism. According to 40–30–30 proponents, lowering blood insulin levels will allow the body to burn fat more efficiently.

*Furthermore, whereas a high-carbohydrate, low-fat meal triggers the release of insulin, a higher percentage of protein will trigger the release of **glucagon**. This hormone has the opposite effect of insulin: it enables the body to burn fat. Therefore, in theory, an athlete who is looking to use more fat for energy during exercise would want to eat less carbohydrate and more protein and fat.*

uct should contain simple and complex carbohydrates, and all of the essential amino acids. Use your supplement strategically to enhance rather than overwhelm your diet and recovery.

Many researchers in sports nutrition, however, have stated otherwise. The fact remains that the consumption of any moderate meal consisting of 60 percent of calories from carbohydrate, 25 percent from fat, and 15 percent from protein, will produce a moderate amount of insulin. The primary role of insulin is to metabolize carbohydrate—not to store fat. Since insulin is busy doing its job on a carbohydrate-rich meal, the concentration of insulin soon falls.

The claim that the 40–30–30 diet helps athletes to lose body fat also remains unproven. This is not because 40–30–30 keeps insulin low in the blood, however. Instead, those who lose body fat are more likely to have done so because they've benefitted from calorie counting to stay within the recommended 2,000-calorie limit. An athlete following the 40–30–30 plan ends up eating less simply because he or she is taking greater care to count calories and to regulate food consumption.

In the end, most nutrition researchers, sports dietitians, and exercise physiologists remain firm in their conviction that the optimal athletic diet consists of 60 percent of calories from carbohydrate, 25 percent from fat, and 15 percent from protein. This recommendation is based on a veritable mountain of validated and convincing research. The experts also advocate supplementing with carbohydrate before and during exercise to improve endurance performance, and consuming carbohydrate after exercise to replenish glycogen stores.

Whey Protein

Whey protein, once thought to be a useless byproduct of cheese production, has recently become one of the most popular protein supplements. This is due, in part, to the development of several methods for distilling whey into a high-quality powder that is fat-and lactose-free. Although it's the most expensive of the three protein powders, whey has a number of advantages over other protein supplements.

One of the greatest benefits of whey protein is that it enhances glutathione production. As you remember from Chapter 8, glutathione is one of the body's natural antioxidants. Therefore, in addition to supplying supplemental protein, whey can help to protect against free-radical damage. Whey protein also has the highest levels of branched-chain amino acids, and it has been shown to boost the immune system. And because whey protein exits the stomach much faster than proteins such as casein, it can be absorbed more quickly into the bloodstream through the intestines. This provides a substantial rise in blood amino acids in a short amount of time, which is important during exercise and recovery. Finally, whey protein dissolves easily in water, making it convenient for a protein drink when you're on the go.

Casein

Casein, another byproduct of cheese production, is included in milk protein powders in varying proportions. Although casein has a higher glutamine content than whey protein, it contains fewer branched-chain amino acids. One disadvantage of milk protein powders is that they don't dissolve easily, so you'll probably need a blender to make your protein drinks. Another concern for some athletes is that casein contains lactose, or milk sugar, which some individuals are unable to digest. Lactose-containing products may cause some people to experience abdominal pain, diarrhea, and excessive gas.

Soy Proteins

Soy proteins, which are high in branched-chain amino

acids and glutamine, were the first protein powders on the market. The isoflavones (plant hormones) in these proteins have been found to exert an estrogenic effect, which can be counterproductive for male athletes. For female athletes, however, the mild estrogenic activity may be beneficial. This is because soy isoflavones can ease menopausal symptoms and promote bone density and other positive effects of estrogen. A disadvantage of soy proteins for both men and women is that they are low in *methionine*, an essential amino acid.

Many soy products require a blender, although newer, top-of-the-line products are easier to mix.

CONCLUSION

Above all else, balanced nutrition is paramount to your success as an athlete because it is crucial to your overall health. Every day, carbohydrate, fat, and protein supply you with energy for your daily activities and help your body to maintain and rebuild tissues. To ensure an adequate intake of these macronutrients, you should consume about 60 percent of calories from carbohydrate, 25 percent from fat, and 15 percent from protein.

Poor nutrition is a nationwide problem. The typical diet, even for active, health-conscious people, often consists of too much saturated fat and a high percentage of simple sugars. On the whole, we need to focus on increasing our intake of the "good" essential fatty acids, while decreasing our intake of processed foods that are high in sugar and low in essential nutrients.

It's important to note that what's considered adequate nutrition for the nonathlete is most likely not adequate to meet your body's requirements. As an active person, you have increased energy needs, so you need to eat more of the energy-yielding macronutrients in the right proportions. You will also want to pay close attention to your protein intake, so that you can counterbalance some of the protein breakdown that occurs during exercise. This may require you to include a protein supplement in your diet in order to meet your elevated requirements.

12.

VITAMINS AND MINERALS: KEYS TO IMPROVED PERFORMANCE

icronutrients are nutrients that are found in the diet and in the body in small amounts. Although we only need trace amounts of these vitamins and minerals, they are essential for optimal performance and, more important, for overall good health. That's because micronutrients often act as *cofactors,* which must be present for other substances in the body to perform their numerous and diverse functions. As cofactors, these nutrients are involved in energy production, oxygen transport, muscle action, and growth. They are also important structural components in your body. And, as you learned in Chapter 8, some vitamins and minerals can act as antioxidants to protect your body from free-radical damage.

Ideally, our diets should supply all of the nutrients we need to meet our daily requirements. But this is the real world. Although we eat some amount of carbohydrates, fats, proteins, and vitamins and minerals every day, the food we consume does not necessarily promote good health. Today, too many of us consume a high percentage of nutrient-poor processed foods, which have lost some of their vitamins and minerals through factors such as freezing, shipping, and storage. Diets that include too much of these foods do not provide the nourishment necessary for optimum health. Instead, they supply the bare minimum of nutrients necessary for survival.

When you exercise, your energy needs increase. Inadequate nutrition, combined with the physical stress of exercise, and on top of life's everyday stresses, may be enough to cause a deficiency of one or several important vitamins and minerals. Therefore, even a diet that is considered to be optimal for a more sedentary person will not be adequate to meet your elevated needs. Like many other athletes, you may find that you benefit from nutritional supplementation.

So how do you know if you are getting enough of the essential vitamins and minerals to ensure your well-being? The tendency, in the past, has been to base the definition of good health on the absence of disease. Clearly, this interpretation is not adequate guidance for the average American, so it's certainly not suitable for an athlete's needs. This chapter begins with a brief outline of the evolution of nutritional guidelines, from the now outmoded Recommended Dietary Allowances (RDAs) to the most recent recommendations for athletes, known as the Performance Daily Intakes (PDIs). You will also find a comprehensive overview of the essential vitamins and minerals that your body requires—not just to prevent deficiency diseases, but to maintain optimum health.

A NEW STANDARD FOR SPORTS NUTRITION

Almost sixty years ago, the National Research Council of the U.S. Department of Health and Human Services recognized the importance of establishing nutritional guidelines for good health. As a result, the Recommended Dietary Allowances (RDAs) were established as the standard for nutrition. In the years following, the NRC periodically published updated RDAs, based upon increasing evidence about nutrient allowances to maintain health.

One of the problems with the RDAs was complexity: for each nutrient, separate recommendations were made based on gender, age, and other factors. By the mid-1980s, scientists and nutritionists disagreed so widely on the recommended allowances that an update was not published for several years. Finally, in 1993, the Nutrition Labeling and Education Act replaced the RDAs with the Reference Daily Intakes (RDIs), which gives the *average* recommendations for twenty-seven vitamins and minerals. By 1997, the RDIs had replaced the RDAs entirely.

The Reference Daily Intakes are not without their own problems, however. For example, like the RDAs, the RDIs represent allowances that are necessary to prevent deficiency. In other words, the RDIs recommend values for essential nutrition for survival—they are not recommendations for amounts that will promote optimum health.

In truth, our bodies need more nutrients and in higher amounts than the RDIs recommend. Nutritionists such as Shari Lieberman, Ph.D., a co-author of *The Real Vitamin and Mineral Book* (Garden City Park: Avery Publishing Group, 1997), have revolutionized the science of nutrition by establishing new guidelines called *Optimum Daily Intakes* (ODIs). These are recommendations for higher allowances of the vitamins and minerals that we require for physical well-being. They take into account the environmental stresses that we encounter every day, as well as the fact that we often don't meet our nutrient requirements through diet alone.

While nonathletes can maintain optimum health by eating balanced meals and supplementing according to the ODI recommendations, athletes must eat a diet that is much more complex. Dr. Kenneth Cooper, a groundbreaker in preventative medicine recognized this need. In *The Antioxidant Revolution* (Nashville: Thomas Nelson Publishers, 1994), Dr. Cooper addresses the need for active people to consume higher amounts of particular vitamins and minerals for protection from serious illnesses.

To help you ensure that you are meeting your requirements for optimum health and maximum athletic performance, I suggest that you follow a new set of standards called the *Performance Daily Intakes* (PDIs). These guidelines were first presented by Daniel Gastelu, M.S., M.F.S., and Fred Hatfield, Ph.D., in their book *Dynamic Nutrition for Maximum Performance* (Garden City Park: Avery Publishing Group, 1997). The PDIs are guidelines for physically active men and women that compensate for the higher nutritional requirements that athletes have over nonathletes.

The remaining sections of this chapter detail the functions and dietary sources of the individual vitamins and minerals. For each nutrient, I have included the recommended Performance Daily Intake, according to the most recent research on the connection between nutrition and performance.

WHAT ARE VITAMINS?

Vitamins are organic compounds that regulate and facilitate the millions of chemical reactions that take place in your body. They do not provide your body with energy in and of themselves, but they do play a role in breaking down and releasing energy from the macronutrients carbohydrate, fat, and protein. Your body cannot make most vitamins, or at least not in substantial amounts, so you have to obtain them from foods or supplements.

The thirteen essential vitamins are divided into two groups. One group consists of fat-soluble vitamins, which the body is capable of storing for weeks or months in the fatty portions of body tissues. The second group consists of water-soluble vitamins, which are found in your body's fluids, and need to be replenished daily because they are rapidly excreted.

The Fat-Soluble Vitamins

Vitamins A, D, E, and K are fat-soluble vitamins that are stored in the liver and fatty tissues until the body needs them. These nutrients require the presence of fats in the diet to be properly digested and absorbed. Therefore, deficiencies are generally reported in individuals who consume diets that are extremely low in fat. Be aware, however, that you need to be especially careful when you supplement with any of these vitamins: when consumed in excess, they have the potential to reach harmful levels in the body because of their storage capabilities.

Vitamin A

Vitamin A is well known for its effectiveness in promoting clear vision and preventing night blindness. It is also needed for cellular growth and development, and for maintaining and repairing all *epithelial tissues*, which make up the skin and internal linings of the respiratory and digestive tracts. Vitamin A functions in the formation of bones and teeth, and it helps to support the immune system, as well. Good sources of vitamin A include liver, fish-liver oil, egg yolks, crab, halibut, whole-milk products, butter, cream, and margarine.

Carotenoids are chemicals found in yellow-red plant pigments that can be chemically converted into vitamin A in the body. The best known of the carotenoids is beta-carotene, which functions as an antioxidant to neutralize free radicals and prevent oxidative damage. Carrots, green leafy vegetables, spinach, broccoli, squash, apricots, sweet potatoes, and cantaloupe are foods rich in beta-carotene.

The PDI of vitamin A is 5,000 to 25,000 IU (International Units). For beta-carotene, the PDI is 15,000 to 60,000 IU for athletes who do not engage in endurance exercise, and 20,000 to 80,000 IU for endurance athletes.

Vitamin D

Vitamin D supports bone formation and maintenance by aiding the body in absorbing calcium and phosphorus, two major structural components of bone tissue. Because of this function, it acts as insurance against rickets, a childhood disease that is characterized by soft, malformed bones, as well as osteoporosis. Vitamin D is believed to improve muscular strength and to enhance immunity, in addition to helping regulate heartbeat.

Vitamin D is found in foods such as eggs, butter, cream, and liver, and seafood, including halibut, herring, mackerel, salmon, sardines, and shrimp. Milk fortified with vitamin D is also a major dietary source.

The Performance Daily Intake of vitamin D is 400 to 1,000 IU.

Vitamin E

As you will remember from Chapter 8, vitamin E is an antioxidant that is important in minimizing free-radical damage. It is also well known for its role in healing wounds because it is a component for normal blood clotting and tissue repair. The maintenance of healthy nerves is another one of vitamin E's many functions.

Dietary sources of vitamin E include soy, corn, cottonseed, peanut, and safflower oils. Vitamin E can also be found in sufficient amounts in dark green leafy vegetables, legumes, nuts, seeds, and whole grains.

The PDI of vitamin E is 200 to 1,000 IU for men and women athletes.

Vitamin K

Vitamin K is essential because it aids in the synthesis of *prothrombin*, a substance that is necessary for blood to clot. The body also uses this nutrient to produce *osteocalcin*, a protein found in large amounts only in bone, and from which calcium is made. Deficiencies of this vitamin are rarely reported because it can be manufactured by the "friendly" bacteria that inhabit the intestines.

The richest sources of vitamin K include green leafy vegetables, asparagus, blackstrap molasses, broccoli, and cabbage. Milk and other dairy products, eggs, cereal, and fruits contain small amounts of vitamin K.

Active men and women will benefit from a PDI of 80 to 180 micrograms (mcg) for vitamin K.

The Water-Soluble Vitamins

Vitamins B_1 (thiamine), B_2 (riboflavin), B_3 (niacin), B_5 (pantothenic acid), B_6 (pyridoxine), B_{12} (cobalamin), and C, as well as folate and biotin are all water-soluble vitamins. The body absorbs these nutrients easily, but because they are quickly excreted in the urine, they are not stored in any significant amount. For this reason, it's important to make sure that you get adequate amounts of the water-soluble vitamins on a daily basis.

Vitamin B Complex

The B complex family of vitamins includes all of the B vitamins, plus folate and biotin. These vitamins are important *coenzymes*, which are cofactors that enable enzymes to carry out their important functions. They help the body to use the macronutrients carbohydrate, fat, and protein to produce energy. Vitamin B_6 functions to help the body use amino acids to manufacture proteins, which are then incorporated into body tissues, used to make hormones, or metabolized for energy. Both vitamin B_{12} and folate aid in cell multiplication, and are necessary for the synthesis of red blood cells, which carry oxygen to other body cells.

Table 12.1 summarizes some of the sources of the B vitamins, as well as the Performance Daily Intake for each vitamin in the B-complex family.

Vitamin C

Vitamin C, or *ascorbic acid,* is probably best known for its roles in preventing the common cold and fighting infec-

Table 12.1. Sources of B-Complex Vitamins

B-Complex Vitamin	Sources	Performance Daily Intake
B_1 (thiamine)	beans, brewer's yeast, peanuts, peas, pork, organ meats, wheat germ	30–200 mg
B_2 (riboflavin)	brewer's yeast, dairy products, fish, fortified grain products, green vegetables, meat, nuts, poultry	30–200 mg
B_3 (niacin)	brewer's yeast, lean meats, legumes, liver, nuts, potatoes, whole grains	20–100 mg
B_5 (pantothenic acid)	beef, eggs, fish, most fruits and vegetables, milk, pork, potatoes, whole wheat	25–200 mg
B_6 (pyridoxine)	bananas, chicken, eggs, fish, kidney, liver, peanuts, rice, soybeans, walnuts	20–100 mg
B_{12} (cobalamin)	beef, clams, eggs, herring, lamb, mackerel, oysters, poultry, tofu	12–200 mcg
Biotin	asparagus, beef, brewer's yeast, eggs, green leafy vegetables, lamb, pork, salmon, whole wheat	125–250 mcg
Folate	brewer's yeast, cauliflower, cereal, egg yolks, legumes, liver, milk, nuts, soy flour	400–1,000 mcg

tions. However, it is also required for the production and maintenance of *collagen,* which is a component of bones, teeth, skin, and tendons. Therefore, it's an important nutrient for the healing of wounds and burns. As an antioxidant, vitamin C helps to minimize free-radical damage.

Because vitamin C cannot be manufactured by the body, it must be obtained from dietary sources or in the form of supplements. Therefore, ensuring adequate intake is very important. Good food sources include citrus fruits, vegetables such as green and red peppers, broccoli, Brussels sprouts, collard greens, spinach, tomatoes, potatoes, and strawberries.

The PDI of vitamin C for athletes is 800 to 3,000 milligrams.

WHAT ARE MINERALS?

Minerals are inorganic nutrients, or nutrients that are not derived from plant or animal matter. They come from the earth's surface, and are absorbed by plants through their roots and incorporated into the structure of the plants. We eventually eat the plants, or the animals that eat plants, and the minerals become part of our own body structure.

Every living cell on this planet depends upon minerals for proper function and structure. Minerals are essential for muscle contraction and the maintenance of healthy nerve function. They also regulate fluid balance, transport substances throughout the body, aid in the formation of blood and bone, and help maintain muscle tone. Like vitamins, minerals enable your body to perform its functions— including energy production—repeatedly and at lightning speed.

Because they are contained in different amounts in the body, minerals are classified according to two groups: the *major,* or macro, minerals; and the *trace,* or micro, minerals. Major minerals are required and contained in your body in larger amounts than are trace minerals. However, both major and trace minerals can cause toxic side effects when they are taken in excessive amounts. Therefore, you should supplement with minerals according to the recommended guidelines, and avoid experimenting with doses that exceed your suggested daily intake.

Major Minerals

The major minerals include calcium, magnesium, phosphorus, and sulfur, as well as the electrolytes chloride, potassium, and sodium. Although magnesium can also function as an electrolyte, it has many nonelectrolyte functions, which we will address specifically in this section.

Major minerals are generally found in the body in amounts larger than 5 grams. Because they are present in larger total quantities, the major minerals influence the body fluids, thereby affecting the whole body in a general way.

Calcium

Calcium is an essential mineral for healthy bone formation and maintenance. In fact, 99 percent of the body's calcium is contained in the bones of the skeleton as *calcium phosphate*. The other 1 percent circulates in blood and other body fluids, and is contained in the body's soft tissues.

Calcium's diverse roles in the body are not limited to the upkeep of bone tissue. For example, it's necessary for muscle growth, as well as the contraction and relaxation of muscles—including the heart. Calcium is also involved in nerve-impulse transmission and blood clotting.

Many of us automatically think of dairy products such as milk, cheese, ice cream, sour cream, cottage cheese, and yogurt as being high in calcium. However, broccoli, kale, collard greens, oysters, shrimp, salmon, and clams are also good sources of calcium that should not be overlooked.

The PDI of calcium for men and women in training is 1,200 to 2,600 milligrams daily.

Special Considerations for Women. Because exercise is known to strengthen existing bone and stimulate the formation of new bone, it is often recommended for women who need to increase bone mass. However, it has been proven that strenuous or long-term exercise can actually have a negative effect on bone density. Surprisingly, increasing numbers of young women athletes actually suffer from a loss of bone mass or thinning of the bone known as *osteoporosis*.

As it turns out, many women who exercise to "lose the fat" may unknowingly lower their body fat to unhealthy levels, below the suggested healthy level of at least 10 percent. Abnormally low body fat interferes with production of the hormone estrogen, which can result in the cessation of menstruation known as *amenorrhea*. And because estrogen is also important in shifting calcium from the bloodstream into the bones, diminished estrogen levels cause the absorption of calcium by the bones to diminish. The end result is that the bones begin to weaken and gradually become brittle.

Unfortunately, simply supplementing with calcium is not the answer to this problem. The bones can only properly absorb calcium when it is in balance with other vitamins and minerals—especially magnesium. In fact, too much calcium can lead to magnesium deficiency. Therefore, women athletes who need to supplement with calcium should take magnesium along with calcium in the proper ratio. Most nutritionists now recommend that the calcium-to-magnesium ratio should be about 2 to 1. Women should also pay particular attention to their intake of several other bone-building nutrients, including vitamins C, D, and K, boron, manganese, and zinc.

Magnesium

In Chapter 6, you learned how magnesium can function as an electrolyte in the body. But magnesium serves many purposes apart from its role as an electrolyte. It is a necessary element in hundreds of enzyme operations, including ATP production for energy. Magnesium also helps to form bones and teeth, and aids in the uptake and balance of two essential minerals for bone development and maintenance, calcium and phosphorus. Researchers have speculated that moderate supplementation with magnesium has the potential to improve endurance and strength for performance. Unfortunately, athletes—in particular, those involved in endurance activities—tend to deplete their magnesium stores, most likely because the body's demand for magnesium increases with an increase in physical activity. Therefore, anyone who exercises would be wise to carefully monitor his or her magnesium intake.

Magnesium can be obtained from dietary sources such as apples, avocados, bananas, brown rice, dairy foods, garlic, green leafy vegetables, legumes, nuts, soybeans, and whole grains.

The PDI of magnesium for healthy, active men and women is 400 to 800 milligrams.

Special Considerations for Women. Women athletes who supplement with calcium in an effort to prevent bone loss are strongly cautioned to monitor their magnesium intake. Remember that calcium and magnesium must be taken in the 2 to 1 ratio to work effectively. When the ratio is exceeded in favor of calcium, magnesium deficiency can sometimes result. This is because increased levels of calcium increase the demand for magnesium to aid in calcium uptake by the bones.

Phosphorus

After calcium, phosphorus is the second most abundant

mineral in the human body. Phosphorus is present in bone as part of calcium phosphate. It is also a component of both adenosine phosphate and creatine phosphate, which store the body's chemical energy. As a constituent of membrane phospholipids, phosphorus functions in maintaining cell membranes, as well. The metabolism of fats and carbohydrates also depend, in part, on the presence of phosphorus.

The best sources of phosphorus are milk, fish, eggs, asparagus, bran, brewer's yeast, corn, legumes, nuts, meats, poultry, salmon, and sesame, sunflower, and pumpkin seeds.

The PDI of phosphorus is 800 to 1,600 milligrams.

Sulfur

Sulfur is part of the chemical structure of many amino acids, including methionine and glutathione. It is found in hemoglobin and in all body tissues, and it is needed for the synthesis of collagen. Sulfur also helps to disinfect the blood, and aids in the body's defenses against toxic substances.

Food sources of sulfur include Brussels sprouts, dried beans, cabbage, eggs, fish, garlic, meats, onions, and soybeans. It is also available in tablet and powder forms.

A Performance Daily Intake has not yet been established for sulfur.

Electrolytes

As we discussed earlier in the book, electrolytes are minerals—including sodium, chloride, and potassium—that conduct the electrical energy of the body, and regulate the flow of water between the cells and the bloodstream. (See page 134 for a discussion of magnesium.) Sodium and chloride are contained mainly in the body's *extracellular fluids*, which are any fluids that are found in the areas of the body outside the cells. Blood and lymph are extracellular fluids. Potassium, on the other hand, is the body's primary *intracellular-fluid* electrolyte, meaning that it is found in the fluids within cells. For a more detailed discussion of the body's major electrolytes, refer to Chapter 6.

The PDI of both sodium and chloride is 1,500 to 4,500 milligrams. Potassium's PDI is 2,500 to 4,000 milligrams.

Trace Minerals

The *trace minerals* include boron, chromium, copper, iodine, iron, manganese, molybdenum, selenium, and zinc. These nutrients occur in the body in smaller amounts than the major minerals, but they are no less important to our survival. Therefore, maintenance of consistent intake is important.

Boron

Boron is a trace mineral that's essential for calcium, phosphorus, and magnesium metabolism, and is therefore important for healthy bone formation. Although some researchers have speculated that boron can increase testosterone production, more research is needed to determine what other benefits it may hold for athletes.

Boron is found in leafy vegetables, fruit, nuts, and legumes. I suggest a daily intake of 5 to 10 milligrams.

Chromium

Chromium aids insulin in the uptake of glucose by muscle cells for energy release. For this reason, a deficiency may result in high blood glucose. There is also evidence that chromium may help lower cholesterol. Furthermore, in the last several years, chromium has received widespread attention as a muscle-builder and fat-burner. Continuing research is necessary before scientists can draw any definite conclusions.

The food sources of chromium include black pepper, brewer's yeast, brown rice, cheese, liver, meat, mushrooms, nuts, potatoes, and whole grains. Chromium is easily processed out of foods, however, so people who eat diets high in refined foods are at risk for chromium deficiency. The PDI of chromium for men and women athletes is 200 to 400 micrograms.

Copper

Copper is an important trace mineral for the formation of *hemoglobin*, the compound in red blood cells that enables them to carry oxygen from the lungs to the tissues via the bloodstream. Collagen requires copper for proper formation, as well. Copper is also present in many enzymes, and is part of the body's natural antioxidant, superoxide dismutase, which helps to protect the body against free-radical damage. Copper has also attracted attention in the sports world for its role in the release of energy.

Nuts, seafood, chocolate, meat, mushrooms, and organ meats—especially liver—are all rich sources of copper. The Performance Daily Intake is 3 to 6 milligrams.

Iodine

Iodine is required for the proper functioning of a gland located in the neck called the *thyroid gland*, which helps regulate metabolism, energy production, growth, and overall physical performance. Iodine deficiency can result in the enlargement of the thyroid, as the cells of the thyroid enlarge to trap as much iodine as possible. The enlargement of the thyroid gland sometimes becomes visible as a lump, which is known as a *goiter.*

Seafood is an excellent source of iodine. Other sources of iodine include iodized salt, spinach, meat, and dairy products. The iodine content of these foods varies depending on the content of the soil in which the plants were grown, or off which animals grazed.

The PDI of iodine is 200 to 400 micrograms.

Iron

Iron is an essential mineral necessary for the formation of the oxygen-carrying compounds hemoglobin and myoglobin. Whereas hemoglobin ferries oxygen from the lungs to the tissues, *myoglobin* carries oxygen within cells. Iron deficiency can result in decreased levels of hemoglobin or myoglobin, which will impair oxygen transport, and ultimately limit exercise performance. When iron intake is low, the body depletes its stores in the bone marrow, spleen, and liver, which can result in the development of anemia.

Iron deficiency can also result from exercise. One possible route for iron loss is *foot-strike hemolysis*. This occurs because some red blood cells are destroyed when the soles of the feet make contact with the hard ground surface. In addition, exercise may cause small blood losses through the digestive tract, at least in some athletes.

Sports anemia is a temporary condition resulting from exercise. Early in training, blood plasma volume increases, which artificially lowers hemoglobin levels. This makes it appear as though an athlete has an iron deficiency. However, sports anemia is not "true" anemia, and it does not impair the oxygen-carrying capacity of hemoglobin. With continued training, sports nutrition disappears on its own.

Iron has recently received attention in the media because of research that links high iron intakes and heart disease. Such reports, however, should not stop people from consuming *adequate levels* of iron. While too much iron may be harmful, too little can negatively affect health and limit athletic performance.

Good dietary sources of iron include meat, poultry, fish, eggs, vegetables, and fortified cereals. Meat sources contain a form of iron known as *heme iron*, which is more readily absorbed by the body than the *non-heme iron* contained in vegetables. In addition, vitamin C has been shown to enhance iron absorption. Also be aware that beverages such as coffee and tea, and the minerals calcium and phosphorus are factors that can hinder iron absorption.

To make sure you're including enough iron in your diet, take a general inventory of the foods you eat, and start checking ingredient lists. It's a good idea to check with your physician before you supplement with iron, so that he or she can make sure that supplementation is absolutely necessary. In addition to getting a standard test for iron, ask for a test of your ferritan levels. *Ferritan* is the storage form of iron. A ferritan test will enable your doctor to tell if your iron stores are adequate.

The PDI of iron for men and women who are actively training is 25 to 60 milligrams.

Special Considerations for Women. Women athletes are especially prone to iron deficiency and anemia for two reasons. First, women lose iron due to blood loss during menstruation. This may cause iron deficiency even without the additional iron losses caused by exercise. Second, studies show that women athletes tend to have low iron intakes. Women on self-imposed calorie-restricted diets, in particular, are at a higher risk for iron deficiency.

Women who suspect that they are iron-deficient are advised to consult a physician for testing before beginning a supplemental regimen. This will pinpoint the cause of iron deficiency, and determine the best course of action to correct the problem.

Manganese

Manganese is a trace mineral that has many important functions for athletes. It is used in energy production, protein and fat metabolism, and bone and connective-tissue formation. The body's natural antioxidant, SOD, is also partly composed of manganese. All of these functions are essential for peak performance.

The richest sources of manganese are avocados, Brussels sprouts, nuts and seeds, seaweed, spinach, turnip greens, wheat germ, and whole grains. For optimum health, active men and women should take in 15 to 45 milligrams of manganese daily.

Molybdenum

Although it is only found in minute quantities in the body, molybdenum is an essential mineral for the maintenance of good health. Molybdenum is a component of several important enzymes that are involved in energy production and nitrogen metabolism.

Dietary sources of molybdenum include milk, beans, cereal grains, legumes, peas, and dark green leafy vegetables.

The PDI of molybdenum for men and women athletes is 100 to 300 micrograms.

Selenium

Selenium is a vital component of the antioxidant enzyme glutathione. The antioxidant activity of selenium is extremely important for athletes because it helps to protect tissues against the oxidative stress of exercise. By minimizing free-radical damage, selenium, in combination with other major antioxidants, can help to reduce recovery time.

As with iodine, the selenium content of a food is dependent upon the selenium content of the soil in which the food is grown. Selenium can be found in varying contents in Brazil nuts, meat, seafood, kidney, liver, and whole grains.

The PDI of selenium is 100 to 300 micrograms.

Zinc

Although it occurs in a very small quantity in the body, zinc plays a role in many metabolic functions. It is part of more than a hundred enzymes that help metabolize carbohydrate, fat, and protein for energy, minimize free-radical damage, and synthesize DNA. Some of these enzymes are also factors in growth and cell replication. Zinc also enhances the actions of vitamin D, which is vital in calcium absorption. And, because it aids in the growth and repair of muscle tissues, zinc is especially important to help athletes recover from the rigors of training.

Meat, whole-grain products, liver, eggs, seafood, herring, oysters, oatmeal, and maple syrup are all known to be food sources rich in zinc.

The Performance Daily Intake of zinc is 15 to 60 milligrams.

CONCLUSION

There's growing evidence that many of us are suffering from some form of micronutrient deficiency. In general, our diets do not provide the nourishment that our bodies require for optimum health. The fact is, the nutritional guidelines that we have followed for more than fifty years provide us only with the recommended *minimum* amounts of vitamins and minerals needed for survival. It's rapidly becoming clear, however, that we should not just eat to survive—we need to take in adequate quantities of vitamins and minerals to help our bodies function at their best.

Obviously, athletes must focus on maintaining optimum health, because an athlete's level of health ultimately determines his or her level of performance. However, physically active people often need more of the essential micronutrients, such as calcium, iron, and the electrolytes, to compensate for the amounts they lose during exercise. At the same time, training requires a high output of energy, which only the increased consumption of nutrients can provide. Fortunately, recent innovations in sports nutrition have resulted in a new set of standards, called the Performance Daily Intakes, to help athletes meet their increased nutritional needs for maximum performance. The PDIs not only provide guidance to help athletes meet their requirements for the hustle and bustle of everyday life—they also ensure maximum nutritional support for the rigors of training and competition.

13.

ENHANCING PERFORMANCE WITH SPORTS SUPPLEMENTS

Have you ever bought and tried a sports nutrition supplement that didn't live up to its claims? Or have you found that, when confronted with an overabundance of sports nutrition products, you simply couldn't decide which would offer the greatest benefits? You're not alone. Faced with manufacturers' competing claims, other athletes also have trouble selecting supplements that will effectively enhance performance.

Because so many of the products available today base their claims on hype, rather than on sound scientific knowledge, it's often very difficult to determine if they can really improve muscle performance—or if they may do more harm than good. To aid you in your quest to select practical, research-proven products, this chapter reviews some of the more popular supplements that have the added benefit of being effective. You'll find that most of these products are available at General Nutrition Centers or your local health foods store.

CAFFEINE

Caffeine is a naturally occurring compound that is found

in coffee, tea, chocolate, cola, and several herbs. Many people use it, in both food form and pill form, as a stimulant or to increase alertness. A good percentage of the population relies on a caffeinated drink to function every morning, or for a boost during the day.

For athletes, however, caffeine is more than just a means to wake up in the morning. Studies have shown that caffeine can also benefit performance. When you exercise, your muscles always use some combination of carbohydrate and fat for fuel. Caffeine increases your body's use of fatty acids for energy, which in turn helps to spare glycogen. It also acts as a nervous-system stimulant to provide a mental boost that helps athletes through strenuous training sessions or long events.

This is all well and good—until we are reminded of caffeine's negative effects on health and, consequently, performance. When you take caffeine in excess—in any form—it can irritate your stomach lining, disrupt sleep, and cause diarrhea. In addition, it acts as a diuretic, which can accelerate dehydration. These are all side effects that you can do without, both in your day-to-day life and during exercise.

If you habitually drink caffeinated coffee or soda, you need to know that you have probably built up a tolerance to caffeine, meaning that you will require greater amounts to see any improvement in performance. To make matters worse, if you are accustomed to daily large amounts of coffee or caffeinated beverages and you try to cut back, you will most likely have to endure withdrawal symptoms before your body can overcome its dependency. Therefore, it's best to use caffeine sparingly, and only periodically, to enhance workouts.

Recommended Dosage

If you do decide to use caffeine to enhance performance

during extended exercise, you'll find that two milligrams per pound of your body weight taken about thirty to sixty minutes before activity may be your optimal dose. For a 160-pound athlete, this means about 320 milligrams before exercise to provide an ergogenic effect. The athlete can obtain this amount from about four 5-ounce cups of brewed (drip method) coffee, each containing 80 milligrams of caffeine. A 5-ounce cup of brewed tea provides 40 milligrams of caffeine, or about half the caffeine of 5 ounces of coffee. Remember that you want to refrain from drinking carbonated beverages such as soft drinks because they can cause gastrointestinal distress. Gas can make you feel full, so that you won't drink as much during and after exercise to rehydrate. If you want a refreshing caffeine-containing drink, you might want to drink iced tea, which contains about 70 milligrams for every 12 ounces.

Do keep in mind, however, that at these levels, caffeine may induce the secretion of stomach acid, which can lead to heartburn. In addition, caffeine's diuretic effect will cause increased water loss through urine in the thirty minutes to two hours after ingestion. This may compound the amount of water that's sweated out during exercise, greatly increasing your chances of dangerous levels of dehydration. As with all things related to nutrition, each individual should evaluate caffeine's effects upon his or her body and consume it at levels that take advantage of its beneficial effects, but minimize the adverse effects of excess intake.

CREATINE

Remember creatine's role in energy production? As we discussed in Chapter 2, your body uses phosphate from creatine phosphate to quickly replenish ATP from ADP. The more energy they store, the better the muscles can perform in events that require explosive power, such as weightlifting, sprinting, jumping, football, hockey, and soccer, to name a few. By consuming creatine, your body can, in effect, make more CP, which will aid in the regeneration of more ATP, enabling your muscles to work at a higher intensity. Creatine can be manufactured by the body, and is also present in food and available in supplemental form.

It's important to note that, so far, only one study has investigated the influence of creatine supplementation on performance in exercise lasting between five and thirty minutes in duration, and there have been no conclusive studies concerning creatine's benefits for exercise lasting more than thirty minutes. Dr. Paul Balsom showed that performance time during a 6-kilometer trail run greater than twenty minutes in duration, was actually impaired after creatine supplementation. This longer running time may have been a result of increased body weight induced by creatine, due to an increase in muscle mass, or simply a reflection of the highly aerobic nature of the exercise task.

The benefits of creatine supplementation for endurance athletes have been heavily researched, especially in the last few years, and have proven that creatine can, in fact, extend endurance. In one study, subjects who were given 20 grams of creatine a day for five days were able to exercise for a significantly longer duration than those who were given a placebo, or fake pill.

Another study showed that creatine supplementation can cause a significant increase in lactate threshold, from 67 percent to 74 percent. This study was conducted with nineteen male and nine female trained runners who ingested 20 grams of creatine a day for seven to eight days. No significant differences were observed in maximal work capacity, however.

One study, completed by Dr. Louise Burke of the Australian Sports Institute, did not show any improvement in swimmers who supplemented with creatine in events such as 25-, 50- and 100-meter sprints. Again, this is likely due to an increase in weight resulting from increased muscle mass. Athletes such as swimmers, who can be slowed down by weight gain, will probably want to avoid supplementing with creatine. Individuals who supplement with creatine monohydrate can expect to increase their weight while decreasing their percentage of body fat, when supplementation is combined with physical training. Endurance athletes are strongly cautioned to avoid putting on too much muscle mass as a result of creatine supplementation because the energy cost of carrying excessive body weight during exercise is increased.

Recommended Dosage

The form of creatine used in all studies showing an ergogenic (performance-enhancing) effect is *creatine monohydrate.* Several quality creatine products are available in capsule and powder form. GNC's Pro Performance Laboratories Creatine Plus, EAS's Phosphagain, and Twin-Lab's Creatine Fuel are good choices for supplementation. A single 5-gram serving of powder is approximately 1 teaspoon. This should be dissolved in some form of liquid directly before consumption.

The best method for increasing and maintaining elevated creatine stores is to start with a five-day loading period, followed by a maintenance period. During the loading phase, a total of 20 to 25 grams of creatine should be taken in 5-gram doses, every two to three hours throughout the day. If you experience any problems, including gastrointestinal problems, when consuming large doses of creatine, you may consider taking 3 grams a day for thirty days during the loading phase.

Since more stored creatine will, together with ATP, produce more energy, it is particularly important to optimize creatine uptake into muscle tissue during this phase. One way of achieving this is to supplement with carbohydrate, which can increase creatine uptake into muscle, and reduce excretion of creatine in the urine. Thus, during the loading phase, carbohydrate should be consumed with the creatine. Once the five-day loading period is complete, the muscles should be fully saturated, which makes further increases unlikely. At this point, maintaining levels of creatine in the muscles becomes an important factor.

A much lower intake of creatine is required to maintain elevated creatine stores. As little as 2 grams a day of creatine will maintain elevated creatine stores in individuals who do not exercise. However, during training, athletes will use more creatine from their stores to resynthesize ATP for energy. In this case, a more appropriate dosage is about 3 to 5 grams a day. In addition, athletes who weigh more than 220 pounds may try taking up to 10 grams a day, because increased muscle mass demands increased levels of creatine.

BETA-HYDROXY BETA-METHYLBUTYRATE

One of today's best-selling anabolic supplements is beta-hydroxy beta-methylbutyrate (HMB). Because HMB is a breakdown product of the amino acid leucine, it aids protein synthesis in the body, which helps to maximize the muscle-building aim of exercise. Although it is found in small quantities in some foods, such as catfish and citrus fruits, athletes may want to supplement with commercial products to secure the full benefits of HMB.

In a study published by Nissen and coworkers, forty-one male volunteers ranging in age from nineteen to twenty-nine, each weighing an average of 180 pounds, were randomly assigned one of two HMB dosages or a placebo. The results showed that subjects gained lean body mass according to the dosage that they had been administered. Total strength for upper- and lower-body exercises increased by an average of 8 percent in subjects who did not supplement. This was compared with an average 13-percent increase in the males taking 1.5 grams of HMB, and 18.4 percent average in subjects who were administered 3 gram-dosages. Researchers also found that subjects who supplemented with HMB were able to lift more weight than subjects who did not supplement during all three weeks. The results of this study clearly indicated that HMB supplementation can improve muscle strength and lean body mass.

The benefits that were apparent with HMB supplementation occurred independently of the level of protein that test subjects consumed. However, it's important to note that even the subjects consuming the least amount of protein were still ingesting large amounts. Therefore, it's possible that a protein intake considered normal by non-bodybuilding standards would limit the benefits of HMB.

Recently, a study conducted by researchers at Iowa State University showed that HMB can also benefit endurance runners. These runners took either HMB or a placebo, in pill form, every day for five weeks. Then, after the fifth week of supplementation, the test subjects ran a 20-kilometer race to test for muscle damage and soreness after exercise. After the race, runners were tested for evidence of muscle damage and loss of strength. The extent of muscle damage was determined by measuring blood levels of creatine phosphokinase, which, as you remember, increases with an increase in muscle damage. The HMB group had significantly lower levels of CPK, meaning that there was less evidence of muscle damage when compared with the placebo group. Measurements of post-race leg strength showed the HMB group lost less muscle strength as well. This study has been the first of its kind to highlight HMB's potential for runners to reduce muscle damage, and to help maintain muscle strength. All of the available research, thus far, has shown HMB to be very beneficial as a muscle builder and protector.

Recommended Dosage

Researchers now recommend supplementation with 3 to 5 grams of HMB per day to build muscle and increase muscle strength. All of the studies to date have shown that HMB is safe and effective for men and women alike. Human studies have been conducted with up to 4 grams of HMB administered daily for up to four weeks. The researchers report no toxicity at these levels. Several HMB products are now available, including EAS's HMB, GNC's Pro Performance HMB, and TwinLab's HMB Fuel.

PHOSPHATIDYLSERINE

Phosphatidylserine (PS), one of the body's phospholipids, is an integral part of the structure and maintenance of cell membranes. Recently, attention has turned to PS as a sports supplement because it can actually help to counteract some of the negative effects of strenuous training. In particular, PS has been shown to reduce the levels of the stress hormone cortisol, which accelerates protein breakdown for energy.

The results of at least three clinical trials have suggested that phosphatidylserine inhibits exercise-induced increases in cortisol. In the first study, investigators found that a 75-milligram dose of PS, when administered intravenously, reduced cortisol release by about 33 percent. Similar results were evident when the study was repeated with 800 milligrams of PS administered in an oral dose. Based on these studies, PS can soften the severity of the body's response to exercise stress.

A recent study by Thomas Fahey, Ed.D., of California State University in Chico, confirmed these results. Eleven college students who trained with weights were given 800 milligrams of oral PS daily and then put through a vigorous, whole-body weight workout four times a week. This regimen was intentionally designed to overtrain the students. Cortisol levels were found to be 20-percent lower in individuals supplementing with PS. Dr. Fahey concluded that up to 800 milligrams of PS is effective in suppressing the cortisol response.

Reducing cortisol has the potential to dramatically improve the way athletes train and use supplements for recovery. Phosphatidylserine can help athletes to recover faster after strenuous workouts by reducing muscle breakdown and the accompanying muscle soreness. It's logical to conclude that PS may even enhance the effectiveness of carbohydrate-protein recovery drinks.

Recommended Dosage

Phosphatidylserine is not available in large quantities in the diet. According to rough estimates, in fact, the total amount of PS that is taken in from food hardly reaches more than 80 milligrams per day. In light of the recent research, athletes may benefit from supplementation to meet the recommended dosage of 400 to 800 milligrams of PS daily.

Until recently, concentrated PS was commercially available only in a bovine-derived product. However, this product was considered to be potentially hazardous because of the threat of mad-cow disease. And safe forms of PS, which were derived from vegetables, only contained trace amounts of the phospholipid. Fortunately, a new form of concentrated PS, which is derived from soybeans, has proven to be a safe, effective source for supplementation. These days, Champion Nutrition markets a brand called Cortistat PS, and GNC sells various PS products made by different manufacturers.

PYRUVATE AND DIHYDROXYACETONE

Pyruvate is the byproduct of carbohydrate metabolism. It

can also be obtained from the diet, with naturally ingested amounts ranging from 100 milligrams to 1 to 2 grams daily. Although pyruvate is found in a variety of foods, most of them contain less than 25 milligrams per serving. Foods high in pyruvate include certain fruits—most notably, red apples—and vegetables, most cheeses, and alcohol products, such as beer and red wine.

Some pyruvate products contain small amounts of *dihydroxyacetone*, which is a compound that can be manufactured by the body and also obtained from the diet. In the body, dihydroxyacetone is rapidly converted during glycolysis to pyruvate. Much of the early research conducted on pyruvate included dihydroxyacetone. The more recent studies have only used pyruvate.

In three studies conducted by Dr. Ronald Stanko at the University of Pittsburgh, pyruvate was shown to improve endurance by enhancing the transport of glucose into the muscles. This process is commonly termed *glucose extraction* because it refers to the amount of glucose extracted by muscles from the circulating blood. A mixture of dihydroxyacetone and pyruvate, known as DHAP, increased glucose extraction by 150 percent after one hour of arm-cycling exercise, and 60 percent for leg-cycling exercise. DHAP also increases glucose extraction when the body is at rest, leading to a possible 50-percent increase in muscle glycogen stores. Research collected from Dr. Stanko's studies also showed that DHAP supplementation over seven days increased endurance in subjects' arms and legs by 20 percent—a very significant increase for athletes. The dosage used in these endurance studies was 100 grams of DHAP, containing 25 grams of pyruvate and 75 grams of dihydroxyacetone.

All of this data suggests that DHAP supplementation can enhance muscle glucose extraction during and after exhaustive exercise. Since glucose is the body's high-energy fuel, increasing glucose extraction for immediate fuel could extend endurance, as well as enhance performance in high-intensity activities such as soccer and basketball. And, of course, enhanced glucose extraction can increase stored energy in the form of muscle glycogen, which will help to extend endurance in subsequent training sessions, or during competition.

Recommended Dosage

According to Dr. Stanko, the most effective dosage of pyruvate is not actually 100 grams a day, but 3 to 5 grams a day, instead. The body does not use pyruvate in excess of these amounts, so results from 10 to 20 grams of pyruvate supplementation will be the same as those seen with 3 to 5 grams.

While the research described above is proof of pyruvate's performance-enhancing effects, it's important to note that these studies were conducted with subjects who did not train regularly. Data has not yet been collected about pyruvate's benefits for well-trained subjects. The preliminary research, however, is enough evidence of the advantages that pyruvate can offer athletes. Some of the better known products on the market are Natural Balance's Pyruvate, GNC's Pro Performance Laboratories Pyruvate, and Bodyonics's Pyruvate 1000.

RIBOSE

When you exercise, some of the ATP that is used for energy is lost from the cell and must be replaced. Recent research has shown that a simple sugar called *ribose* can actually stimulate the body's production of ATP. Ribose is an essential molecule for ATP production and maintenance in the heart and skeletal muscles.

Ribose production in the heart and skeletal muscles, however, is a slow process that cannot keep up with this loss of energy during intense exercise. Under conditions of maximal exercise, there is a substantial decrease in the total ATP pools in skeletal muscle cells, and it may take several days to completely replace the energy molecules that are lost. In fact, the results of studies have indicated that decreases in these nucleotides can be as much as 20 percent to 28 percent after periods of high-intensity exercise.

Skeletal muscles are very efficient at conserving energy, but when they are called upon to perform maximum work, the number of energy producing or energy conserving molecules that are lost can be significant. As long as there is a sufficient amount of oxygen present in the cell for aerobic metabolism, muscle cells are able to recycle energy virtually without losing any ATP molecules. However, during periods of very hard physical work, when there is not enough oxygen absorbed into the bloodstream to supply the demand of the cells, a large percentage of the total pool of ATP can be lost. Because there is no known food source that supplies a sufficient amount of ribose to be metabolically significant, ribose supplementation is essential to quickly replace ATP used by the cell.

A considerable amount of research has been done to show that the loss of ATP by skeletal muscle can be severe during periods of intense exercise. In one study, eleven healthy male volunteers underwent six weeks of high-intensity training three times per week followed by one week with two training sessions per day. A second group of nine healthy volunteers did not exercise for the first six weeks, but trained twice a day along with the first group during the final week.

The results showed that ATP levels in the thigh muscles of the first group dropped 13 percent during the six weeks of training. ATP levels in the muscle tissues of this group did not go down further during the final week of training. This shows that after a period of intense exercise, ATP dropped to well below pre-training levels. More significant, however, is the fact that even after three days of rest following the last exercise bout, ATP levels in this first group still did not recover to pre-training levels. In fact, ATP in the muscle cells of these subjects were still almost 10 percent below their pre-training levels. In other words, even after this three-day rest period the thigh muscles were not able to fully replace their lost ATP.

In the second group, the effect was even more dramatic. This group did not have a period of training before beginning high-intensity exercise in the final week. Instead, the subjects went from being sedentary to performing two exercise bouts per day for one week. In this group, ATP in thigh muscle dropped by 25 percent immediately after the last exercise bout. Even after three days of rest, this group still had an ATP pool that was 19.5 percent less than it had initially.

Recommended Dosage

Research has shown that about 3 to 5 grams of ribose taken every day should put enough in the blood to be sure that heart and skeletal muscle cells have an adequate supply. I suggest starting out with about 5 grams of ribose per day. If you feel you need more, increase at about 2 to 3 grams per day, but it should not take more than 15 to 20 grams per day to get the positive effects ribose gives. If you are in serious physical training, you may want to take up to 10 grams per day to start. If you are not in training, but just want to maintain healthy levels of energy in your heart and skeletal muscles, 3 to 5 grams per day should be an adequate maintenance dose.

CONCLUSION

In today's sports world, it's becoming increasingly popular for athletes to use natural supplements to optimize recovery and enhance performance. By increasing the rate of energy production and replenishment, protecting against muscle damage, and maximizing muscle building, these products may be just what some athletes need to gain that extra competitive edge. However, misconceptions about the relationship between certain supplements and exercise performance can lead athletes to expect unrealistic results. Researchers are still gathering information about the benefits—and possible side effects—of many of these cutting-edge products.

In any case, it's important to keep the benefits of sports supplements in the proper perspective. Products such as creatine and ribose should be incorporated into your regular training schedule to enhance recovery and performance, rather than being used alone. As always, it's best to do your homework, and to remain informed of the latest research on the products you choose.

14.

NUTRITION TO DELAY EVENT FATIGUE

While training and post-exercise nutrition are essential for consistent performance, what you eat—and how much of it you eat—in the days and hours before competition is just as important in delaying fatigue. One of the most popular and effective nutritional methods for delaying the fatigue brought on by low glycogen stores is to first deplete the body's glycogen stores, and then consume a high-carbohydrate diet in the days prior to your event. This technique is known as *carbohydrate loading* or *glycogen supercompensation*.

During regular training, an athlete should consume a proportion of nutrients that contains approximately 60 percent of calories from carbohydrate, 25 percent from fat, and 15 percent from protein. Starting a few days before competition, however, endurance athletes who carbo load will boost their carbohydrate intake to up to 70 percent of dietary calories. This chapter discusses the nutritional basis for carbohydrate loading, and presents two effective methods for achieving exceptional results.

CARBOHYDRATE DEPLETION AND REPLENISHMENT

During the 1970s, researchers studied the effects of diets containing various levels of carbohydrate on performance during intensive exercise. They found that when subjects exercised intensely to deplete their glycogen stores, and then consumed a carbohydrate-rich diet each day for several days afterwards, their endurance was significantly increased.

As you will remember from earlier chapters, your muscles use carbohydrate as their primary source of energy during intensive exercise. Whatever is not used is transported to the muscles and liver, where it is stored as glycogen for future use. When your body needs energy, glycogen stores are converted back to glucose, and burned as fuel. Even though glycogen is your body's most important source of energy, your body's capacity to store glycogen is limited. When you have used most or all of the available glycogen supply, your body begins to break fat down into fatty acids for energy. In addition, during long-term exercise, some of the amino acids that make up muscle tissue are used to fuel your body's activity, which negatively affects your efforts to build up muscle tissue.

Carbohydrate loading helps to ensure that your glycogen stores will not be so quickly depleted during exercise. Carbo loading also enables your muscles to store glycogen more efficiently, so that when you enter the days of high-carbohydrate feedings, your muscles become supercompensated with glycogen.

WHO BENEFITS FROM CARBOHYDRATE LOADING?

Carbohydrate loading is a useful tool for helping athletes to avoid "hitting the wall," so, in general, endurance athletes reap the greatest benefits from this dietary regimen. These athletes include long-distance swimmers, cross-country skiers, soccer players, long-distance runners (especially marathoners), triathletes, and long-distance cyclists. For the most part, any athlete participating in an event lasting more than ninety minutes will find carbo loading to be highly effective. While it is unlikely that you will hit the wall in an event lasting less than ninety minutes, such as a basketball or a football game, or a track-and-field event, you may still find carbo loading to be moderately beneficial. Just try tapering off training a few days before competition, and boosting the percentage of carbohydrate in your diet.

You should be aware that some athletes should not practice carbohydrate loading at all. Athletes who need to meet weight-class requirements should avoid carbo loading because of the high caloric intake during the days preceding competition. Other athletes state that they feel bloated, or that their muscles feel "heavy" after a week of a high-carbohydrate diet and reduced training, and they complain that this hinders, rather than enhances, their performance. This is because, for every gram of carbohydrate that you store, you also store between 3 and 5 grams of water. If you are considering carbohydrate loading before an important competition, you should make a trial run before a minor competition, or during the off-season to see how your body responds.

There have not been any consistent reports of long-term gains in body weight with fluctuating glycogen levels. Any weight that an athlete puts on from carbo loading is most likely due to water weight gain. Interestingly enough, there may actually be an advantage to gaining this water weight before competition: extra water can be used to help cool you down by allowing for sweating during high-intensity exercise in the heat.

METHODS OF CARBOHYDRATE LOADING

There are two general methods of carbohydrate loading that are considered to be effective. The first method was

Fat Loading for Endurance?

Recently, some individuals have advocated the practice of "fat loading" to spare glycogen stores and increase endurance. The reasoning behind this is that fat is your body's most energy-rich nutrient, containing 9 calories in one gram. (Calories are units used to measure food energy.) Therefore, when compared with carbohydrate, which has only 4 calories in a gram, fat is shown to contain more than twice the energy.

So why haven't endurance athletes started eating cookies for breakfast, or munching potato chips for a pre-exercise energy boost? The most obvious reason seems to be that, from a nutritional standpoint, a diet loaded with refined, processed foods that are high in the "wrong" kinds of fats is a health disaster waiting to happen. Pertaining to sports, high-fat diets have been shown to actually reduce glycogen stores, and, as a result, to impair performance. In one study, individuals ate a diet consisting of 76-percent fat for four days. After the fourth day, when the subjects were asked to run until exhaustion, those who had fat loaded

built upon the early research on glycogen depletion and replenishment, and includes very intense training in the days prior to competition. The second method is a modified version of the first regimen, and has proved to be less stressful on the body, but equally effective.

The Classical Regimen

The *classical regimen* of carbohydrate loading became very popular in the 1970s. This technique requires you to complete intense training sessions for three days and maintain *reached exhausion 40 percent sooner than those who had consumed a diet lower in fat.*

The reason for this is that the body can't oxidize fat as well as it can glycogen during intense exercise. During exercise, only about 30 percent of your body's energy is derived from fat. And even though fat may produce more energy per gram, your body needs about 75 percent more oxygen to "burn" the fat. This puts greater stress on your cardiorespiratory system.

When all's said and done, exhaustion during exercise is still directly linked to glycogen depletion. Therefore, to forestall exercise-induced fatigue, you should eat a high-carbohydrate diet during training. If you train at high intensity, you should include about 3 to 5 grams of carbohdyrate in your diet per pound of your body weight. If you have difficulty achieving this goal, you might find it beneficial to use a carbohydrate supplement before, during, and after training to load, sustain, and replenish glycogen stores. Also, be sure to use the guidelines presented in this chapter for carbohydrate loading prior to any competition lasting longer than ninety minutes.

a low-carbohydrate diet in order to deplete your body's glycogen stores. Following the three-day depletion phase is a three-day period during which you should consume a diet that includes 70 percent of calories from carbohydrate and you should cut back on training intensity. The classical regimen has been shown to increase a trained athlete's muscle glycogen stores by two to two and a half times, which results in extended endurance.

This method of carbo loading does have drawbacks, however. Some athletes are not comfortable training to exhaustion four or five days before competition. Many also find that training becomes difficult when glycogen stores are at such low levels because they simply have less energy. As a result, the quality of the athlete's workout suffers, leaving some competitors feeling that they are not properly prepared for their events. In addition, low glycogen stores can lead to fatigue and improper form, which increases the risk of injury.

The Modified Regimen

Fortunately, Dr. Michael Sherman of Ohio State University has shown that glycogen supercompensation can be achieved through the *modified regimen* for carbo loading. This method has been shown to raise glycogen levels comparably to the levels induced by the classical regimen—with few side effects. Dr. Sherman recommends that, during the six days before competition, athletes consume a 50-percent carbohydrate diet for three days, followed by a 70-percent carbohydrate diet for three days before competition. During this six-day period, exercise duration is progressively decreased from ninety minutes on the first day, to about forty minutes on the second and third days, to approximately twenty minutes on the fourth and fifth days, to very light exercise or total rest on the final day. This regimen is outlined in Table 14.1 on page 163.

But how do you know that you are obtaining the proper percentage of carbohydrate from your diet? One way is to go by percentage of total caloric intake. You can also consume 2 grams of carbohydrate for every pound of your body weight a day during the 50-percent days, and up to 5 grams of carbohydrate for every pound of body weight a day during the 70-percent days.

BOOSTING YOUR CARBOHYDRATE INTAKE

If you've ever tried to maintain a diet that includes a large

Table 14.1. Modified Regimen for Carbohydrate Loading

Day	Exercise Duration	Percent of Calories From Carbohydrates
1	90 minutes	50%
2	40 minutes	50%
3	40 minutes	50%
4	20 minutes	70%
5	20 minutes	70%
6	Rest	70%
7	Race	70%

percentage of calories from carbohydrate, you know that it's no easy task! Remember that, gram for gram, carbohydrate contains less than half the calories of fat. You may want to use high-carbohydrate drinks to supplement your carbohydrate intake. These will allow you to consume large amounts of carbohydrates without the added bulk.

Whichever regimen you choose to follow, keep in mind that all kinds of carbohydrate can help replenish glycogen stores. However, before a training session, those with low glycemic indexes work best because they release glucose into the bloodstream slowly, allowing for a steady release of carbohydrate into your bloodstream. (For a discussion of glycemic indexes, see the inset in Chapter 7.)

In addition, try to increase your portions of complex carbohydrates. Foods such as cereals, pasta, breads, grains, and beans will provide you with vitamins, minerals, fiber, and protein, as well as carbohydrate. Try to stay away from simple sugars, since they tend to be low in vitamins, minerals, and fiber. The rest of your diet should contain foods that are good sources of protein and fat.

CONCLUSION

Haphazard eating habits in the days before competition

can sabotage any athlete's performance. At some point, almost all athletes encounter obstacles during competition that they cannot overcome, such as decreased endurance, difficulty concentrating, and reduced strength. In most cases, these are problems that could have been prevented or minimized with proper pre-competition nutrition.

Competition places special demands on your body above and beyond those of training, and you must be physically prepared to meet those demands. The starting point is sound nutritional knowledge and practice. Carbohydrate loading is a valuable means to forestall fatigue and perform at peak capacity during long events. But keep in mind that carbo loading is not a daily nutritional regimen for performance and, as such, it should be practiced only when necessary about a week before competition. When your event is not close at hand, you should rely on carefully balanced nutrition for overall health and optimal recovery.

15.

NONNUTRITIONAL APPROACHES TO RECOVERY

It has been said that the race is not always to the swift, but to those who keep on training. Throughout this book, we have focused on the nutritional strategies that you can use to make the most of your recovery from exercise. As the previous chapters have shown you, the R^4 System—in combination with nutritional supplementation and natural sports products—will enable you to "keep on training" by helping you to maximize recovery and minimize muscle soreness.

Still, it would be unrealistic to believe that any nutritional program could entirely do away with muscle damage or soreness. In light of this, our guidelines for recovery would not be complete without a discussion of some nonnutritional methods that can provide relief for your hardworking muscles. For example, relaxation in a sauna or hot tub can be very therapeutic for post-exercise aches and pains. Sports massage is also an incredible recuperative tool because it helps to eliminate the physical and psychological effects of fatigue, as well as to reduce the risks of muscle injury. And simple stretching exercises during warm-up and cool-down periods are a must in keeping muscles strong and flexible, and preventing damage to muscle tissue.

MASSAGE

Sports massage is not a new concept in Europe. In fact, a great number of European athletes incorporated this technique into their regular training and competition schedules long ago, and continue to appreciate its merits today. Although athletes in North America have generally been hesitant to accept massage as an integral part of training, more and more active men and women are beginning to sample the benefits for themselves.

Chris Carmichael, coach to professional cyclist Lance Armstrong, has stated that "Prior to and during major competitions, without massage and competent medical care, many athletes I've worked with would not have done as well. [Massage] relaxes the muscles, particularly after heavy training when they feel completely spent. It helps them relax and fully recover."

Researchers at the Karolinska Institute in Stockholm also found evidence to support the beneficial effects of massage. In this study, a group of competitive cyclists pedaled to exhaustion, and then had a ten-minute rest period. Half of the group received ten-minutes of massage while they rested, while the other half did not receive massage. After the rest period, all of the subjects were asked to do fifty knee extensions on an exercise machine that tested leg strength. The researchers found that leg quadriceps muscles were 11-percent stronger in the cyclists that had received massage therapy when compared with the cyclists that had rested for ten minutes.

Whether it is administered before or after exercise, to soothe away muscle soreness or to help maintain overall muscle health, there's no doubt that massage offers positive benefits for almost every athlete. Let's first take a look at how massage helps to maintain overall muscle health.

Muscle Maintenance

When incorporated into an athlete's training schedule, massage is said to promote recovery from intense training schedules, as well as to increase training potential. Regular massage promotes the health of hardworking muscles by improving the circulation of body fluids and by preventing blood from pooling in the capillaries of muscles. Improved circulation also enhances the exchange of substances between blood and tissue cells. In addition, massage helps to decrease swelling in muscle tissues, and to stretch and relax sore, overworked muscles—all of which alleviate pain.

Although massage does not directly increase normal muscle strength, it is more effective than rest in promoting recovery from the soreness and fatigue brought on by excessive training or competition. It helps keep your muscles in the best possible state of health and flexibility, so they can function at maximum potential even after recovery from hard exercise.

Pre-Competition Massage

Preparatory massage before competition increases or decreases the excitability of the nerve cells—depending on the type, duration, and intensity of the massage. In addition, supporters of massage say that it warms the muscles, joints, and ligaments, helping to keep them loose and flexible. This protects against injury to cell membranes, also known as *microtrauma*.

Pre-competition massage focuses on stretching and warming up the ligaments and tendons of the arms and legs. Because these connective tissues don't have their own blood supply, they don't warm up as quickly as muscle tissue. Massage helps to improve circulation, which results in increased blood flow to relaxed muscle tissues. This, in turn, results in enhanced blood flow to tendons and ligaments. An added benefit is that massage given prior to competition exerts a purely psychological effect by helping anxious and tense athletes to calm down.

It's best to begin pre-competition massage before the warm-up period. Slow stroking can be used to calm the athlete, while a kneading, tapping, or vibrating stroke should stimulate and warm the muscles. The massage should be followed by stretching and a normal, comprehensive warm-up session.

Post-Competition Massage

Most athletes who have experienced post-competition massage will tell you that nothing feels better when the day is done. The therapist works systematically on the athlete's body, progressing from feet, legs, lower back up to the shoulders until all the knots and kinks have been worked out. As the muscles relax and loosen, they become more pliable, enhancing the state of relaxation.

Massage therapy following competition helps to eliminate the effects of muscle fatigue. It relieves sore and tense muscles, to some extent, while maintaining flexibility and elasticity in the muscles, tendons, and ligaments. Restorative massage after competition is said to speed muscle recovery two to three times faster than just resting, because it promotes blood flow, which works to carry nutrients and oxygen to muscles for repair, and to carry byproducts of metabolism away from muscles.

Hard exercise causes microtrauma to occur in cells, along with some swelling of the muscle tissues. Massage can help to minimize these consequences, or at least to alleviate any pain that accompanies them. Usually, a combination of deep longitudinal strokes to stimulate blood flow; jostling or shaking to relax the muscles; and cross-fiber massage, which involves rubbing across the muscle, is used to relieve pain and stiffness, and to smooth out trigger points that have flared up due to training or racing.

Allow at least thirty minutes after a hard race for a thorough massage in order to feel fully recovered—physically as well as psychologically. The massage should be given in the evening, about one to one and a half hours after your evening meal. This will leave time for the meal to be partially digested so that blood flow—which is greater to the stomach during digestion—can be directed to the muscles.

Injury Repair

Massage can be beneficial in providing a greater range of muscle movement in injured athletes, and it can also help to speed healing at the site of the injury. In addition, it has a positive psychological effect by relaxing and soothing the athlete, thereby reducing the emotional stress that comes with inactivity.

Despite the benefits of massage, however, Andy Pruitt, Certified Athletic Trainer and Director of Sports Medicine at the Boulder Center for Sports Medicine, advises caution in implementing massage therapy if the athlete has sustained muscle damage. "Massage will only traumatize the injured area further under these conditions," says Pruitt. Therefore, massage should not be applied to injured tissue for forty-eight to seventy-two hours after the initial trauma, and certainly not until the swelling and pain have substantially subsided. The three main contraindications to massage [for injured muscles only] are deep muscle trauma, surface abrasions, and tendinitis.

With the increased blood and lymph movement, massage increases nutrition to joints and muscles while hastening the reduction of swelling and the elimination of accumulated inflammatory waste products. The primary ways that lymph moves through the body is through deep breathing, muscular movement, or massage. Massage pressure can help stimulate the lymphatic vessels when exercise is impossible. It is also beneficial in maintaining muscle tone and delaying muscular atrophy, which may result from time off from training.

SAUNAS

Many aching athletes have experienced the soothing and relaxing benefits that a session in a *sauna,* or steam bath, can provide. The heat and moisture of the sauna induce perspiration, which helps to cleanse the body of impurities through sweating, and relieve aches and pains by speeding up circulation and raising body temperature. While the virtues of the sauna as a miracle treatment may be exaggerated, there is scientific and medical evidence that points to its legitimate beneficial effects.

An early study done by Dr. Herb de Vries at the University of Southern California found that the heat of a sauna relaxes muscles. Dr. de Vries measured the electrical activity in the muscles of several subjects who were taking a sauna. He found that the sauna's heat actually brought about a significant decrease in muscle tension. For the competitive athlete, a reduction in muscle tension encourages relaxation, promotes speedy recuperation, and enhances an overall sense of physical and emotional well-being.

The humid heat of the sauna has also been found to help eliminate some of the byproducts of metabolism. During a long hard exercise session, an athlete may experience a breakdown of tissue protein to be used for fuel, which increases the body's nitrogen level. Nitrogen is a byproduct of protein breakdown that the body cannot use. It is usually removed from the blood by the kidneys and then excreted in the urine. However, a sauna hastens the elimination of nitrogen through the skin as well. Using a sauna allows a faster recovery from the long training and strenuous training sessions because the kidneys do not have to work as hard to eliminate excess nitrogen.

Research has also shown that repeated sessions in the sauna can be as effective as regular mild exercise in conditioning the cardiovascular system. And, in addition to its countless other benefits, the sauna can aid in acclimation to heat stress. The heat of the sauna stresses the body's cooling mechanisms, and this gradually improves the body's capacity to withstand heat. This is important if you are from a cooler region, and are preparing for an event that is to take place in a warmer climate. You can increase your body's ability to function in the heat, so that you'll be ready to compete when you arrive.

A popular misconception about saunas is that they are effective tools for weight loss. While you may burn some calories due to the increased demands put on your body by the heat, any significant drop in body weight is only due to water loss. A few glasses of water after a session will put you right back up in weight.

A few words of caution: If you are pregnant, or if you have heart disease or high blood pressure, it's important to consult your physician before you begin taking saunas. This is because the sauna can increase your heart rate. Also, delay your sauna session if you have the symptoms of any illness. The sauna's heat will place added stress on your body, which is already stressed due to the illness. Finally, don't drink alcoholic beverages immediately before or during a session in the sauna. Alcohol has a diuretic effect, which may increase the risk of dehydration.

To derive the greatest possible benefit from a session in the sauna, take note of the following guidelines:

❑ Allow plenty of time to ensure a leisurely session for maximum benefit. Divide your session into several shorter intervals with a brief rest period in between each. Also allow time for a longer rest period after you are through.

❑ Start with moderate heat, and adjust the temperature when you learn at which point your body is most comfortable.

❑ To start with, sit or lie down on the lowest shelves at the start of each session, where the air is cooler. From there you can work your way up to the higher shelves for more intense results.

❑ Allow at least twenty minutes for the last cooling down period; this should include a shower. If possible, don't towel off immediately; but let the air dry your skin as you cool off. Some people experience lightheadedness and extreme fatigue after a sauna. After resting, however, these sensations should dissipate.

❑ Replace fluids after your session in order to bring your body back to its normal state of hydration.

Traditional electric heat saunas use the convection system, which heats up the air in order to heat up your body. These systems require between thirty and sixty minutes to preheat so the moisture in the air is evaporated, and the internal temperature is allowed to rise to the proper range of 180 to 200°F. Recently, there has been an increase in the sales of saunas that use a radiant form of heat, which heats up the body directly, rather than first heating the air. Radiant heat saunas are more efficient and economical, requiring only ten to fifteen minutes to preheat, and a few cents per hour to operate. Radiant heat saunas allow your body to perspire at lower temperatures of about 105 to

130°F. This type of sauna is more comfortable, so you'll be able to extend the length of your sessions.

STRETCHING

While watching the coverage of the Tour de France last year on television, I noticed that a commentator remarked on the fluid pedaling movements of experienced cyclists such as Jan Ullrich and Bobby Julick. The announcer was amazed by their ability to pedal effortlessly, even while they took time to stretch their shoulders, lower back and legs while cycling in the breakaway.

After thousands of training miles, professional cyclists have learned techniques to reduce the minor aches and pains that can result from sitting on their bikes in long road races. But stiff, sore muscles are not the bane of cyclists alone. Any athlete who trains long and hard is especially prone to "exercise rigor mortis," a gradual loss of muscle elasticity, accompanied by an increase in joint stiffness. Therefore, athletes have found it necessary to develop simple stretching techniques that allow them to perform at their maximum capacity, while reducing tightness and pain in the lower back, shoulders, neck, face, arms, feet, and legs.

As you ride, row, swim, or strength-train on resistance equipment, your muscles become stronger, but tighter— and this tightness can lead to muscle pain. This is a warning sign that you are experiencing a gradual loss of muscle elasticity and a decrease in joint flexibility. Stretching, which requires no special skill and relatively little time, can help prevent stiff and sore muscles, and aid in recovery.

Stretching before your workout will help blood to circulate through your muscles, which will warm them up. This warm-up period increases nutrient flow to tissues, and provides a period of adjustment to prepare muscles for the hard work to come. Stretching between exercises, or when you change pieces of equipment, can relieve muscle tension and postpone fatigue. In addition, stretching after your workout should be part of your comprehensive cooldown period to ensure muscle relaxation, and prevent muscle soreness. Stretching in the post-exercise period also helps to circulate nutrients to muscle tissues, and to carry waste products away from the muscles. Best of all, stretching exercises done at any time before, during, or after exercise, will help you to maintain flexibility, which decreases your risk of muscle injury, and increases your physical efficiency and performance.

Stretching Techniques

A long, sustained stretch known as a *static stretch* is a far superior method of stretching your muscles and the surrounding connective tissue when compared with a *ballistic stretch*, which is a rapid and uncontrolled bouncing stretch. Ballistic stretching is generally not recommended for the general population because the high force and short duration of this technique can increase the risk of injury.

You should get used to the feeling of an easy static stretch that's low in intensity and that lasts for fifteen to thirty seconds. A static stretch will cause a slight pulling sensation in the muscle, but it *should not be painful.* If you stretch correctly, and maintain the easy stretch for enough time, the result will be less tension in the muscles you are stretching.

Stretching Exercises

Figures 15.1 through 15.3 show a general ten-minute program that can be done before, after, or even during your workout. These same stretches can also be used during the competition season to aid with stiffness you may experience after a long, hard workout session.

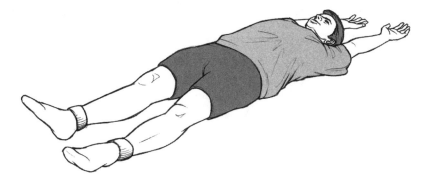

Figure 15.1. Elongation

Straighten out your arms and legs. Point your fingers and toes as you stretch as far as you can. Hold for five seconds, then relax. This is a good way to stretch your entire body.

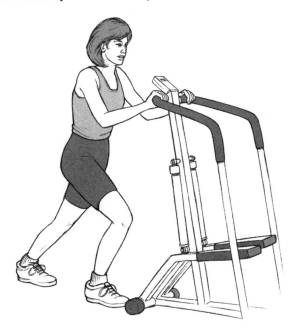

Figure 15.2. Achilles and Calf Stretch

Your back leg should start out straight with the foot flat and pointing straight ahead. Then bend your back knee slightly, still keeping your foot flat. This gives you a much lower stretch, which is good for maintaining or regaining ankle flexibility. Hold for fifteen seconds for each leg. Do not strain the muscles too much—this area needs only a slight sensation of stretching.

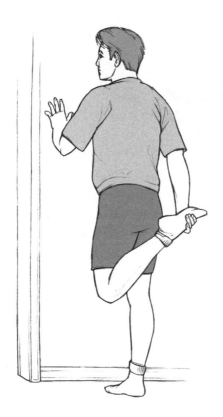

Figure 15.3. Standing Quads
Hold the top of your left foot (on the inside) with your right hand and gently pull the heel toward your buttocks. Repeat with your left hand holding your right foot.

Figure 15.4. Shoulder Shrug
Raise the top of your shoulders toward your ears until you feel slight tension in your neck and shoulders. Hold your shoulders at this point for three to five seconds, and then relax your shoulders downward into their normal position. Do this two to three times. This technique is good to use at the first signs of tightness or tension in the shoulder and neck area.

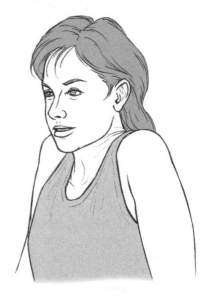

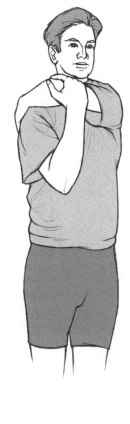

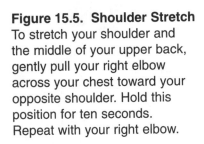

Figure 15.5. Shoulder Stretch
To stretch your shoulder and
the middle of your upper back,
gently pull your right elbow
across your chest toward your
opposite shoulder. Hold this
position for ten seconds.
Repeat with your right elbow.

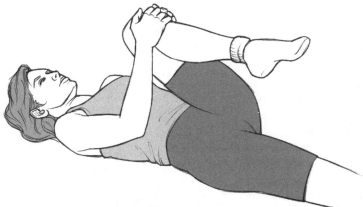

Figure 15.6. Williams Flex Stretch
Straighten both legs and relax, then pull your right leg toward your
chest. For this stretch, keep the back of your head on the mat, if
possible, but do not strain. Repeat with your left leg.

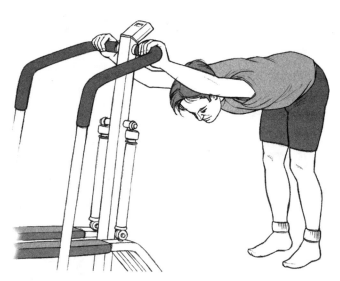

Figure 15.7. Fence Pull

Place both hands shoulder width apart on a ledge and let your upper body drop down as you keep your knees slightly bent. Your hips should be directly above your feet. To change the area of the stretch, bend your knees just a bit more and/or place your hands at different heights. This will take some of the kinks out of a tired upper back.

Figure 15.8. Groin Stretch

Put the soles of your feet together with your heels a comfortable distance from your groin. Then, holding your feet with your hands, slowly pull yourself forward until you feel an easy stretch in the groin. Make your forward movement by bending from the hips, not from the shoulders.

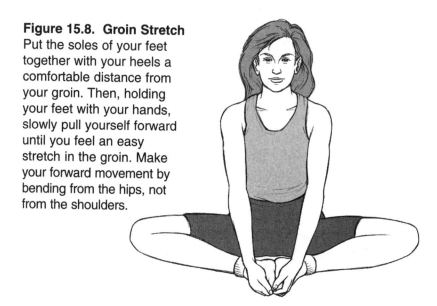

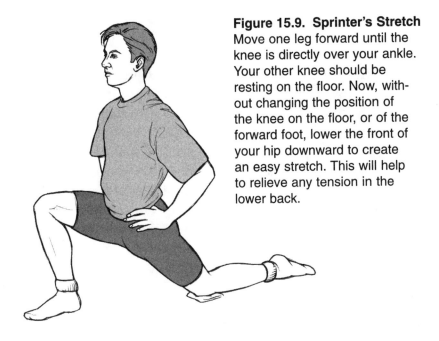

Figure 15.9. Sprinter's Stretch
Move one leg forward until the knee is directly over your ankle. Your other knee should be resting on the floor. Now, without changing the position of the knee on the floor, or of the forward foot, lower the front of your hip downward to create an easy stretch. This will help to relieve any tension in the lower back.

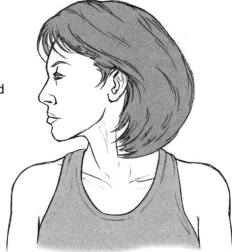

Figure 15.10. Neck Stretch
From a stable, aligned sitting position, turn your chin toward your right shoulder to stretch the left side of your neck. Hold correct stretch tensions for ten to twenty seconds. Stretch each side twice.

CONCLUSION

Nonnutritional approaches to recovery are as important to overall fitness and muscle recovery as strength and aerobic conditioning. These days, it's not uncommon for athletes to depend on a thorough massage to warm up their muscles before competition, or for total body relaxation after an event or training session. Many athletes have also discovered that relaxing in a sauna can work wonders on tired, aching muscles. The heat and moisture of the sauna have been proven to speed up circulation, which increases the flow of vital nutrients to damaged or inflamed muscle tissues. And, in addition to helping the body recover from exercise, these methods double as valuable relaxation time, which is beneficial to emotional health and well-being.

Whether or not you make time for a massage or a session in the sauna, you should *always* stretch properly before and after exercise. Just a few minutes of simple stretching exercises prior to exercise can help enhance circulation so that your muscles will be warmed up and ready for action. After exercise, stretching ensures proper muscle relaxation, and keeps blood flowing at an increased rate to transport nutrients to fatigued and damaged muscle tissues.

CONCLUSION

The secret to reaching a high level of performance cannot be found in any one food or supplement. Nor does it lie in pushing your body beyond its capacity day after day. *Optimal Muscle Recovery* has shown you, in just a few short chapters, what it has taken many top athletes years to discover: peak performance depends upon optimal recovery from exercise.

In the last few years, the importance of allowing for recovery time as part of regular training has really come to the forefront. It has been reflected in the design of workout sessions that are less frequent and of shorter duration. Athletes are also being advised to make time for adequate sleep, and to take measures to reduce day-to-day stresses. Now, cutting-edge research points to nutrition as an essential piece of the recovery puzzle.

The R^4 System is based on fascinating research that has significantly advanced our understanding of muscle physiology. It incorporates the latest information concerning the need to restore fluids and electrolytes, both during and after exercise. Rehydration is, in fact, the cornerstone of the R^4 System, because sufficient fluid balance is absolutely critical in order to support the body's cardiovascular function and to regulate body temperature. Studies have proven that electrolytes are key factors in facilitating fluid absorption to minimize dehydration.

Powerful evidence pinpointing insulin's role as the master recovery hormone has been collected from studies conducted at leading universities. These studies have highlighted the importance of consuming key nutrients—most notably, carbohydrate and protein—in the proper proportions within the first two hours after exercise. This stimulates insulin to "kick start" the body's glycogen replenishment and muscle repair processes.

Scientists and nutritionists have also discovered a connection between strenuous exercise and the buildup of free radicals in the body. Experts now advocate supplementation with antioxidants, including vitamins C and E, in order to minimize free-radical damage, thereby shortening recovery time. Related research into the effects of exercise stress has shown that intense activity compromises the immune system, as well, making athletes more susceptible to colds and infections. Natural substances such as glutamine, ciwujia, and even carbohydrate can keep the immune system—and, therefore, the athlete—strong and healthy.

It has been my intention to provide you with some insight into the basic science of recovery, in order to give you a head start on improving your individual performance. Although the principles of the R[4] System have grown out of mountains of highly technical scientific evidence, the guidelines for recovery remain simple and practical enough for every athlete to incorporate into training.

Meeting your body's energy needs after exercise will give you the strength and endurance you need to reach your long-term goals for training and competition. Your workout doesn't stop when you get off your bike, take off your running shoes, or walk out of the gym. You're not finished until you have refueled and followed the guidelines of the R[4] System to ensure optimal muscle recovery.

GLOSSARY

Actin. The protein that forms the thin filaments in a muscle fiber.

Adenosine diphosphate (ADP). The molecule formed when one of the phosphate molecules is removed for energy production in the cell.

Adenosine triphosphate (ATP). The source of energy for all living cells.

ADP. *See* Adenosine diphosphate.

Aerobic metabolism. Metabolism in the cell that takes place in the presence of oxygen.

Amino acids. The "building blocks" of proteins. There are 20 different amino acids used by the body.

Anaerobic metabolism. Metabolism in the cell that takes place when there is not sufficient oxygen supplied by the blood to maintain aerobic metabolism.

Antioxidants. Nutrients that seek out and neutralize free radicals in the body, and help the body to recovery more quickly from free-radical damage.

ATP. *See* Adenosine triphosphate.

ATP-CP pathway. One of the two anaerobic energy pathways. Energy is released when adenosine triphosphate (ATP) loses one phosphate molecule and becomes adenosine diphosphate (ADP). Creatine phosphate (CP) donates phosphate to replenish ATP stores.

Ballistic stretch. A rapid and uncontrolled bouncing stretch; generally not recommended because of the risk of injury.

Branched-chain amino acids. Amino acids that supply energy by taking the place of glucose in energy pathways; leucine, isoleucine, and valine.

Calories. Units used to measure food energy.

Carbohydrate loading. A nutritional method for delaying fatigue in which the athlete depletes his or her glycogen stores, and then consumes a high-carbohydrate diet in the days prior to a competitive event; also known as glycogen supercompensation.

Cardiac muscle. The type of muscle that is found only in the heart.

Central fatigue. Fatigue that results from impaired function of the central nervous system; mental fatigue.

Cofactor. A substance that must be present for another substance to be able to perform a particular function.

Complete proteins. Proteins that contain all of the nine essential amino acids.

Complex carbohydrates. Carbohydrates that are composed of long chains of glucose molecules.

Cortisol. A hormone that's released in response to all kinds of stress, including psychological, physical, and emotional stresses.

Creatine phosphate (CP). A molecule in the cell that serves as an energy-producing component.

Creatine phosphokinase (CPK). A biochemical marker that is a measure of muscle damage.

Dehydration. The condition caused by excessive loss of water from the body.

Electrolytes. Mineral salts that conduct the electrical energy of the body, and are responsible for muscle contraction and nerve-impulse transmission; sodium, chloride, magnesium, and potassium.

Enzymes. A protein that promotes a chemical reaction without itself being altered in the process.

Ergogenic aid. A nutritional supplement that enhances muscular strength or performance.

Essential amino acids. Those amino acids that the body cannot manufacture, and that must be supplied by the diet.

Essential fatty acids. Fatty acids that are necessary for rebuilding and producing new cells, and maintaining proper brain and nervous-system function.

Fast-twitch muscle fibers. Muscle fibers that contract quickly, providing short bursts of energy; used when strength and speed are needed.

Fatty acids. Components of fat molecules that are used to produce energy.

Foot-strike hemolysis. A condition that occurs because red blood cells are destroyed when the soles of the feet make contact with the hard ground surface.

Free radical. An atom or molecule that is short one electron. It actively seeks out and steals electrons from other parts of the cell.

Glucose. A simple sugar that supplies the body with immediate fuel for energy.

Glutamine. An amino acid that functions as a source of energy for immune cells, and is also readily available for the synthesis of skeletal muscle proteins.

Glycemic index. A measure of the effect of carbohydrate on blood glucose levels.

Glycogen. A chain of glucose molecules; the form in which glucose is stored in the liver and muscle tissues; it is broken down into glucose for energy when needed.

Glycogen supercompensation. *See* Carbohydrate loading.

Glycogen synthase. An enzyme in the muscle cells that is responsible for converting glucose into glycogen for storage.

Gram (g). A unit of weight. One pound equals 454 grams.

Hemoglobin. The protein responsible for transporting oxygen to muscle cells.

Incomplete proteins. Proteins that are missing one or more of the essential amino acids.

Insulin. A hormone released by the pancreas that helps glucose enter cells from the blood.

International Unit. A unit of weight, usually used for fat-soluble vitamins.

Lactate threshold. The point at which the level of lactic acid in the blood is greater than the body can metabolize.

Lactic acid. A byproduct of anaerobic metabolism that cannot be used effectively by working muscles.

Macronutrients. Nutrients that the body requires daily in large amounts to function properly; water, carbohydrate, fat, and protein.

Microgram (mcg). A unit of weight. A microgram is one-millionth of a gram, or one-thousandth of a milligram.

Micronutrients. Nutrients that are found in the diet and in the body in small amounts; vitamins and minerals.

Microtrauma. Injury to cell membranes.

Milligram (mg). A unit of weight. A milligram is one-thousandth of a gram.

Mitochondria. The structures within cells that are the sites of aerobic energy production.

Myofibrils. The units of muscle fibers that are directly involved in contraction.

Myoglobin. The protein responsible for delivering oxygen from the cell membrane to the mitochondria.

Myosin. The protein that forms the thick filaments in a muscle fiber.

Nonessential amino acids. Amino acids that can be manufactured by the body from other amino acids, and therefore do not have to come from the diet.

Osteoporosis. Loss of bone mass or thinning of the bone.

Oxidation. A reaction in which an atom loses an electron.

Rehydration. The process of restoring fluid volumes.

Simple carbohydrates. Carbohydrates that consist of single glucose molecules.

Skeletal muscle. The muscles that cause the movement of bones, also known as voluntary muscle and striated muscle.

Slow-twitch muscle fibers. Muscle fibers that produce a slow, low-intensity, repetitive contraction and are therefore used for long-term exercise.

Smooth muscle. The type of muscle tissue found in the organs of the digestive system and the walls of blood vessels; also known as involuntary muscle.

Sports anemia. A temporary condition resulting from the increase of blood plasma volume, which artificially lowers hemoglobin levels.

Static stretch. A long, sustained stretch that last for fifteen to thirty seconds.

Tryptophan. An amino acid that is essential for human metabolism. Tryptophan can cause sleepiness and fatigue when it enters the brain.

REFERENCES

Chapter 1: How Muscles Work

Belanger, A.Y. and A.J. McComas. "A comparison of contractile properties in human arm and leg muscles." *European Journal of Applied Physiology* 54 (1985): 26–33.

Campbell, C.J., et al. "Muscle fiber composition and performance capacities of women." *Medicine and Science in Sports* 11 (1979): 260–265.

Essen, B.E., et al. "Metabolic characteristics of fibre types in human skeletal muscle." *Acta Physiolgica Scandinavica* 19 (1975): 153–165.

Gollnick, P.D., et al. "Effect of training on enzyme activity and fiber composition of human skeletal muscle." *Journal of Applied Physiology* 34 (1973): 107–111.

Green, J.F. and A.P. Jackman. "Peripheral limitations to exercise." *Medicine and Science in Sports and Exercise* 16 (1984): 299–305.

Chapter 2: The Energy Currency of Muscles

Chang, T. Wen and A.L. Goldberg. "The metabolic fates of amino acids and the formation of glutamine in skeletal muscle." *Journal of Biological Chemistry* 253 (1978): 3685–3695.

Conzolazio, C.F., et al. "Protein metabolism during intensive physical training in the young adult." *American Journal of Clinical Nutrition* 28 (1975): 29–35.

DiPrampero, P.E. "Energetics of muscular exercise." *Biochemical Pharmacology* 89 (1981): 143–209.

Holloszy, J.O. "Adaptation of skeletal muscle to endurance exercise." *Medicine and Science in Sports* 7 (1975): 155–164.

Karlsson, J. and B. Saltin. "Lactate, ATP, and CP in working muscles during exhaustive exercise in man." *Journal of Applied Physiology* 29 (1970): 598–602.

Jacobs, I., et al. "Sprint training effects on muscle myoglobin, enzymes, fiber types, and blood lactate." *Medicine and Science in Sports and Exercise* 19 (1987): 369–374.

Chapter 3: What Causes Fatigue?

Ahlborg, B., et al. "Muscle glycogen and muscle electrolytes during prolonged physical exercise." *Acta Physiologica Scandinavica* 70 (1967): 129–142.

Buono, M.J., T.R. Clancy and J.R. Cook. "Blood lactate and ammonium ion accumulation during graded exercise in humans." *The American Physiological Society* (1984): 135–139.

Brouns, F. *Nutritional Needs of the Athlete* (Chichester, Great Britain: John Wiley & Sons, 1993).

Brilla, LR. and K.B. Gunter. "Effects of magnesium supplementation on exercise time to exhaustion." *Medicine, Exercise, Nutrition and Health* 4 (1995): 230–233.

Costill, D.L., et al. "Muscle water and electrolyte distribution during prolonged exercise." *International Journal of Sports Medicine* 2 (1981): 130–134.

Costill, D.L. and M. Hargreaves. "Carbohydrate nutrition and fatigue." *Sports Medicine* 13 (1992): 86.

Costill, D.L., et al. "Effects of repeated days of intensified training on muscle glycogen and swimming performance." *Medicine and Science in Sports and Exercise* 20 (1987): 249–254.

Coyle, E.F. and A.R. Coggan. "Effectiveness of carbohydrate feeding in delaying fatigue during prolonged exercise." *Sports Medicine* 5 (1984): 446–458.

Davis, JM. "Carbohydrate, branched-chain amino acids and endurance: The central fatigue hypothesis." Gatorade Sports Science Institute *Sports Science Exchange* 9 (1996): 1–6.

Davis J.M. and S.P. Bailey. "Possible mechanisms of central nervous system fatigue during exercise." *Medicine and Science in Sports and Exercise* 29 (1996): 45–57.

Konig, D., et al. "Zinc, iron, and magnesium status in athletes—Influence on the regulation of exercise-induced stress and immune function." *Exercise and Immunology Review* 4 (1998): 2–21.

Murray, R., et al. "The effect of fluid and carbohydrate feedings during intermittent cycling exercise." *Medicine and Science in Sports and Exercise* 19 (1987): 597–604.

Neiman, D.C. "Influence of carbohydrate on the immune response to intensive, prolonged exercise." *Exercise Immunology Review* 4 (1998): 64–76.

Newsholme, E.A. "Psychoimmunology and cellular nutrition: An alternative hypothesis." *Biological Psychiatry* 27 (1990): 1–3.

Nose, H., et al. "Shift in body fluid compartments after dehydration in humans." *Journal of Applied Physiology* 65 (1988): 318–324.

Rudolph, D.L. and E. McAuley. "Cortisol and affective responses to exercise." *Journal of Sport Sciences* 16 (1998): 121–128.

Chapter 4: What Causes Muscle Soreness?

Armstrong, R.B. "Mechanisms of exercise-induced delayed onset muscular soreness: A brief review." *Medicine and Science in Sports and Exercise* 16 (1984): 529–538.

Armstrong, R.B. "Muscle damage and endurance events." *Sports Medicine* 3 (1986): 370–381.

Armstrong, R.B., G.L. Warren, and J.A. Warren. "Mechanisms of exercise induced muscle fiber injury." *Sports Medicine* 12 (1991): 184–207.

Evans, W.J. and J.G. Cannon, ed. J.O. Holloszy. *The Metabolic Effects of Exercise-induced Muscle Damage in Exercise and Sport Sciences Reviews* (Baltimore, MD: Williams & Wilkins, 1991), pp. 99–126.

Kanter, M. "Free radicals, exercise, and antioxidant supplementation." *International Journal of Sport Nutrition* 4 (1994): 205.

Round, J.M., D.A. Jones, and G. Cambridge. "Cellular infiltrates in human skeletal muscle: Exercise-induced damage as a model for inflammatory muscle disease?" *Journal of Neurological Sciences* 82 (1987): 1–11.

Warholt, M.J., et al. "Skeletal muscle injury and repair in marathon runners after competition." *American Journal of Pathology* 118 (1985): 331–339.

Chapter 5: Recovery: Your Key to Peak Performance

Thomas, D., et al. "Plasma glucose levels after prolonged strenuous exercise correlate inversely with glycemic response to food consumed before exercise." *International Journal of Sport Nutrition* 4 (1994): 361.

Hofman, Z., et al. "Glucose and insulin responses after commonly used sport feedings before and after a 1-hour training session." *International Journal of Sport Nutrition* 5 (1995): 194–205.

Hermansen, L., E. Hultman, and B. Saltin. "Muscle glycogen during prolonged severe exercise." *Acta Physiolgica Scandinavica* 71 (1967): 129–139.

Chapter 6: Restore Fluid and Electrolytes

Buchman, A.L., C. Keen, J. Commisso, et al. "The effect of a manathon run on plasma and urine mineral and metal concentrations." *Journal of the American College of Nutrition* 17 (1998): 124–127.

Maughan, R.J. "Fluid and electrolyte loss and replacement in exercise." *Journal of Sports Sciences* 9 (1991): 117–142.

Murray, R. "The effects of consuming carbohydrate-electrolyte beverages on gastric emptying and fluid absorption during and following exercise." *Sports Medicine* 4 (1987): 322–351.

Nose, H.G., et al. "Role of osmolality and plasma volume during rehydration in humans" *Journal of Applied Physiology* 65 (1988): 325–321.

Rehrer, N.J., et al. "Effects of electrolytes in carbohydrate beverages on gastric emptying and secretion." *Medicine and Science in Sports and Exercise* 25 (1993): 42–51.

Chapter 7: Replenish Glycogen Rapidly

Ahlborg, B., et al. "Muscle glycogen and muscle electrolytes during prolonged physical exercise." *Acta Physiologica Scandinavia* 70 (1967): 129–142.

Bergstrom, J., et al. "Diet, muscle glycogen and physical performance." *Acta Physiologica Scandinavia* 71 (1967): 140–150.

Biolo, G., et al. "An abundant supply of amino acids enhances the metabolic effect of exercise on muscle protein." *American Journal of Physiology* 273 (1997): E122–E129.

Blom, P.C.S., et al. "Effect of different post-exercise sugar diets on the rate of muscle glycogen synthesis." *Medicine and Science in Sports and Exercise* 19 (1987): 491–496.

Burke, L.M., G.R. Collier, and M. Hargraves. "Glycemic index— A tool in sport nutrition." *International Journal of Sport Nutrition* 8 (1998): 401–415.

Burke, L.M., G.R. Collier, and M. Hargreaves. "Muscle glycogen storage after prolonged exercise: effect of the glycemic index of carbohydrate feedings." *Journal of Applied Physiology* 75 (1993): 1019–1023.

Copinschi, G., et al. "Effect of arginine on serum levels of insulin and growth hormone in obese subjects." *Metabolism* 16 (1967): 485–491.

Costill, D.L., et al. "Muscle and liver glycogen resynthesis following oral glucose and fructose feedings in rats." *Biochemistry of Exercise,* Vol. 13, eds. H. Knuttgen, J. Vogel and J. Poortmans (Champaign, IL: Human Kinetics, 1983), pp. 281–285.

Ivy, J.L., et al. "Muscle glycogen storage after different amounts of carbohydrate ingestion." *Journal of Applied Physiology* 65 (1988): 2018–2023.

Ivy, J.L., et al. "Muscle glycogen synthesis after exercise: Effect of time of carbohydrate ingestion." *Journal of Applied Physiology* 64 (1988): 1480–1485.

Reed, M.J., et al. "Muscle glycogen storage postexercise: Effect of mode of carbohydrate administration." *Journal of Applied Physiology* 66 (1989): 720–726.

Roy, B.D., et al. "Effect of glucose supplement timing on protein metabolism after resistance training." *Journal of Applied Physiology* 82 (1997): 1882–1888.

Sherman, W.M., et al. "Dietary carbohydrate, muscle glycogen, and exercise performance during 7 days of training." *American Journal of Clinical Nutrition* 57 (1993): 27–31.

Spiller, G.A., et al. "Effect of protein dose on serum glucose and insulin response to sugars." *American Journal of Clinical Nutrition* 46 (1987): 474–480.

Tarnopolsky, M.A., et al. "Postexercise protein-carbohydrate and carbohydrate supplements increase muscle glycogen in men and women." *Journal of Applied Physiology* 83 (1997): 1877–1883.

Varnier, M., et al. "Stimulatory effect of glutamine on glycogen accumulation in human skeletal muscle." *American Journal of Physiology* 269 (1995): E309–E315.

Yarasheski, K.E., J.J. Zachwieja, and D.M. Bier. "Acute effect of resistance exercise on muscle protein synthesis rate in young and elderly men and women." *American Journal of Physiology* 265 (1993): E210–E214.

Zawadzki, K.M., B.B. Yaspelkis, and J.L. Ivy. "Carbohydrate-protein complex increases the rate of muscle glycogen storage after exercise." *Journal of Applied Physiology* 72 (1992): 1854–1859.

Chapter 8: Reduce Muscle and Immune Stress

Adibi, S.A. "Intravenous use of glutamine in peptide form: Clinical applications of old and new observations." *Metabolism* 38(supplement 1) (1989): 88–92.

Bowles, D.K., et al. "Effects of acute, submaximal exercise on skeletal muscle vitamin E." *Free Radical Research Communication* 14 (1991): 139–143.

Byrnes, W.C., et al. "Delayed onset muscle soreness following repeated bouts of downhill running." *Journal of Applied Physiology* 59 (1985): 710–715.

Cannon, J.G., et al. "Acute phase response in exercise. Associations between vitamin E, cytokines, and muscle proteolysis" *American Journal of Physiology* 260 (1991): R1235–R1240.

Cannon, J.G., et al. "Acute phase response in exercise: Interaction of age and vitamin E on neutrophils and muscle enzyme release." *American Journal of Physiology* 259 (1990): R1214–R1219.

Castell, L.M., et al. "The role of glutamine in the immune system and in intestinal function in catabolic states." *Amino Acids* 7 (1994): 231–243.

Castell, L.M., J.R. Poortmans, and E.A. Newsholme. "Does glutamine have a role in reducing infection in athletes?" *European Journal of Applied Physiology* 73 (1996): 488–490.

Davies, K.J.A., et al. "Free radicals and tissue damage produced by exercise." *Biochemical and Biophysical Research Communications* 107(4) (1982): 1198–1205.

Gleeson, M., J.D. Robertson, and R.J. Maughan. "Influence of exercise on ascorbic acid status in man." *Clinical Science* 73 (1987): 501–505.

Gohil, K., et al. "Vitamin E deficiency and vitamin C supplements: Exercise and mitochondrial oxidation." *Journal of Applied Physiology* 60 (1986): 1986–1991.

Handbook of the Composition and Pharmacology of Common Chinese Drugs (Beijing: Chinese Medical Technology Press, 1994), p. 1186.

Hartmann, A., et al. "Vitamin E prevents exercise-induced DNA damage." *Mutation Research* 346 (1995): 195–202.

Hikida, R.S., et al. "Muscle fiber necrosis associated with human marathon runners." *Journal of Neurological Sciences* 59 (1983): 185–203.

Hiscock, N. and L.T. Mackinnon. "A comparison of plasma glutamine concentrations in athletes of various sports." *Medicine and Science in Sports and Exercise* 30 (1998): 1693–1696.

Jacob, R.A. and B.J. Burri. "Oxidative damage and defense." *American Journal of Clinical Nutrition* 63 (1996): 985S–990S.

Kaman, R. *Endurox: A Novel Agent That Increases Workout Performance* (Woodbridge, NJ: PacificHealth Laboratories Inc.).

Keast, D., et al. "Depression of plasma glutamine concentration after exercise stress and its possible influence on the immune system." *Medical Journal of Australia* 162 (1995): 15–18.

Lawrence, J.D., et al. "Effects of atocopherol acetate on the swimming endurance of trained swimmers." *American Journal of Clinical Nutrition* 28 (1975): 205–208.

Lehmann, M., C. Foster, and J. Keul. "Overtaining in endurance athletes: A brief review." *Medicine and Science in Sports and Exercise* 25 (1993): 854–862.

McBride, L.M., et al. "Effect of resistance exercise on free radical production." *Medicine and Science in Sports and Exercise* 30 (1998): 67–72.

Meydanit M., et al. "Muscle uptake of vitamin E and its association with muscle fiber type." *Journal of Nutritional Biochemistry* 8 (1997): 74–78.

Meydanit, M., et al. "Protective effect of vitamin E on exercise-induced oxidative damage in young and older adults." *American Journal of Physiology* 264 (1993): R992–R998.

Neiman, D.C. "Influence of carbohydrate on the immune response to intensive, prolonged exercise." *Exercise Immunology Review* 4 (1998): 64–76.

Newsholme, E.A. "A biochemical mechanism to explain some characteristics of overtraining." *Advances in Nutrition and Topics in Sport* 32 (1991): 79–93.

Newsholme, E.A. "Psychoimmunology and cellular nutrition: An alternative hypothesis." *Biological Psychiatry* 27 (1990): 1–3.

Newsholme, E.A. and M. Parry-Billings. "Properties of glutamine release from muscle and its importance for the immune system." *Journal of Parenteral* 14 (1990): 635–675.

Parry-Billings, M., et al. "Communicational link between skeletal muscle, brain and cells of the immune system." *International Journal of Sports Medicine* 11(special supplement) (1990): 1–7.

Quintanilha, A.T. and L. Packer. *Vitamin E, Physical Exercise and Tissue Oxidative Damage in Biology of Vitamin E* (London: E. Pitman, 1983), pp. 56–69.

Robertson, J.D., et al. "Increased blood antioxidant systems of runners in response to training load." *Clinical Science* 80 (1991): 611–618.

Rohde, T., K. Krzywkowski, and B.K. Pedersen. "Glutamine, exercise, and the immune system—Is there a link?" *Exercise Immunology Review* 4 (1998): 49–63.

Rokitai, L., et al. "Alpha-tocopherol supplementation in racing cyclists during extreme endurance training." *International Journal of Sport Nutrition* 4 (1994): 253–264

Rowbottom, D.G., et al. "The hetematological, biochemical and immunological profile of athletes suffering from the overtraining syndrome." *European Journal Applied Physiology* 70 (1995): 502–509.

Rowbottom, D.G., D. Keast, and A.R. Morton. "The emerging role of glutamine as an indicator of exercise stress and overtraining." *Sports Medicine* 21 (1996): 80–97.

Scaglione, F., et al. "Immunomodulatory effects of two extracts of *Panax ginseng*." *Drugs Exptl Clinical Research* 16 (1990): 537–542.

Sharman, I.M., M.G. Down, and N.G. Norgan. "The effects of vitamin E on physiological function and athletic performance of trained swimmers." *Journal of Sports Medicine* 16 (1976): 215–225.

Sharman, I.M., M.G. Down, and N. Sen. "The effects of vitamin E and training on physiological function and athletic performance in adolescent swimmers." *British Journal of Nutrition* 26 (1971): 265–276.

Shephard, R.J., et al. "Vitamin E, exercise and the recovery from physical activity." *European Journal of Applied Physiology* 33 (1974): 119–126.

Simon-Schnass, I. and H. Pabst. "Influence of vitamin E on physical performance." *International Journal of Vitamin and Nutrition Research* 58 (1988): 49–54.

Stone, M.H., R.E. Keith, J.T. Kearney, et al. "Overtraining: A review of the signs, symptoms and possible causes." *Journal of Applied Sport Sciences Research* 5 (1991): 35–50.

Walsh, N.P., et al. "Glutamine, exercise and immune function." *Sports Medicine* 26 (1998): 177–191.

Chapter 9: Rebuild Muscle Protein

Davis, J.M.. "Carbohydrate, branched-chain amino acids, and endurance: The central fatigue hypothesis." *International Journal of Sport Nutrition* 5 (1995): S29–S38.

Davis, J.M. "Carbohydrate, branched-chain amino acids and endurance: The central fatigue hypothesis." Gatorade Sports Science Institute *Sports Science Exchange* 9(2) (1996): 1–6.

Davis, J.M. and Bailey S.P. "Possible mechanisms of central nervous system fatigue during exercise." *Medicine and Science in Sports and Exercise* 29 (1996): 45–57.

Johnson, D.J., Z.M. Jiang, M. Cotpoys, et al. "Branched-chain amino acid uptake and muscle free amino acid concentrations predict postoperative muscle nitrogen balance." *Annals of Surgery* 204 (1986): 513–523.

Johnson, D.J., Z.M. Jiang, M. Cotpoys, et al. "Branched-chain amino acid uptake and muscle free amino acid concentrations predict postoperative muscle nitrogen balance." *Annals of Surgery* 204 (1986): 513–523.

Kreider, R.B., V. Miriel, and E. Bertun. "Amino acid supplementation and exercise performance: An analysis of the proposed ergogenic value." *Sports Medicine* 16 (1993): 190–209.

Lemon, P.W.R. "Do athletes need more dietary protein and amino acids?" *International Journal of Sport Nutrition* 5 (1995): S39–S61.

Madsen, K., et al. "Effects of glucose and glucose plus branched-chain amino acids or placebo on bike performance over 100 km." *Journal of Applied Physiology* 81 (1996): 2644–2650.

Newsholme, E.A., I.N. Acworth, and E. Blomstrand. "Amino acids, brain nerotransmitters and a functional link between muscle and brain that is important in sustained exercise." *Advances in Myochemistry*, ed. G. Benzi (London: John Libbey Eurotext, 1989), pp. 127–133.

Chapter 10: Making Science Practical: The R^4 System Drink

Ready, S.L., J. Seifert, and E. Burke. "Effects of two sport drinks on muscle stress and performance." Abstract presented at National Meeting of the American College of Sports Medicine, 1999.

Williams, M., J. Ivy, and P. Raven. "Effects of recovery drinks after prolonged glycogen-depletion exercise." Abstracts presented at Mid-Atlantic Regional Meeting, 1998, and National Meeting of the American College of Sports Medicine, 1999.

Chapter 11: Nutrition for Every Day

Coleman, E. "The BioZone nutrition system: A dietary panacea?" *International Journal of Sport Nutrition* 6 (1996): 69–71.

Golay, A., et al. "Similar weight loss with low- or high-carbohydrate diets." *American Journal of Clinical Nutrition* 63 (1996): 174–178.

"Higher fat 40/30/30 diet fad." American Running and Fitness Association *Running & Fitness News,* 14(8) (1996): 1.

Karlsson, J., and B. Saltin. "Diet, muscle glycogen, and endurance performance." *Journal of Applied Physiology* 31 (1971): 203–206.

Lemon, P.W.R. "Effects of exercise on protein requirements." *International Journal of Sport Nutrition* 8 (1998): 426–447.

Sears, B. *The Zone* (New York, NY: Harper Collins, 1995), pp. 40–54.

Sherman, W. and N. Leenders. "Fat loading: The next magic bullet?" *International Journal of Sport Nutrition* 5 (1995): S1–S12.

Young, K., and C.T.M. Davies. "Effect of diet on human muscle weakness following prolonged exercise." *European Journal of Applied Physiology* 53 (1984): 81–85.

Young, V.R. and P.L. Pellett. "Protein intake and requirements with reference to diet and health." *American Journal of Clinical Nutrition* 45 (1987): 1323–1343.

Chapter 12: Vitamins and Minerals: Keys to Improved Performance

Brilla, LR. and K.B. Gunter. "Effects of magnesium supplementation on exercise time to exhaustion." *Medicine, Exercise, Nutrition and Health* 4 (1995): 230–233.

Cooper, K.H. *Advanced Nutritional Therapies* (Nashville, TN: Thomas Nelson Publishers, 1996).

Cooper, K.H. *Antioxidant Revolution* (Nashville, TN: Thomas Nelson Publishers, 1994).

Gastelu, D. and F. Hatfield. *Dynamic Nutrition for Maximum Performance* (Garden City Park, NY: Avery Publishing Group, 1997).

Karlson, J. *Antioxidants and Exercise* (Champaign, IL: Human Kinetics Publishers, 1997).

Kies, C.V. and J.A. Driskell. *Sports Nutrition: Minerals and Electrolytes* (Boca Raton, FL: CRC Press, 1995).

Konig, D., et al. "Zinc, iron, and magnesium status in athletes—Influence on the regulation of exercise-induced stress and immune function." *Exercise and Immunology Review* 4 (1998): 2–21.

Lieberman, S. *The Real Vitamin and Mineral Book* (Garden City Park, NY: Avery Publishing Group, 1997).

Ulene, A. and V. Ulene. *The Vitamin Strategy* (Berkeley, CA: Ulysses Press, 1994).

Wolinsky, I. *Nutrition in Exercise and Sport* (Boca Raton, FL: CRC Press, 1998).

Wolinsky, I. and J.A. Driskell. *Sports Nutrition* (Boca Raton, FL: CRC Press, 1997).

Chapter 13: Enhancing Performance With Sports Supplements

Abumrad, N. and P. Flakoll. "The efficacy and safety of HMB (Beta-hydroxy-Beta-methylbutyrate) in humans." Vanderbilt University Medical Center, Annual Report: MTI, 1991.

Alamada, A., T. Mitchell, and C. Earnest. "Impact of chronic supplementation on serum enzyme concentrations." *FASEB Journal* 10 (1996): A4567.

Almada, A., et al. "Effects of B-HMB supplementation with and without creatine during training on strength and sprint capacity." *FASEB Journal* 11(3) (1997): A374.

Balsam, P., et al. "Creatine supplementation per se does not enhance endurance exercise performance." *Acta Physiologica Scandinavia* 149 (1993): 521–523.

Balsom, P.D., K. Soderlund, and B. Ekblom. "Creatine in humans with special reference to creatine supplementation." *Sports Medicine* 18(4) (1994): 268–280.

Burke, E. *Creatine: What You Need to Know* (Garden City Park, NY: Avery Publishing Group, 1999).

Burke, E. *D-Ribose: What You Need to Know* (Garden City Park, NY: Avery Publishing Group, 1999).

Burke, E. and T. Fahey. *Phosphatidylserine: Promise for Athletic Performance* (New Canaan, CT: Keats Publishing, 1998).

Burke, E. *Pyruvate* (New Canaan, CT: Keats Publishing, 1997).

Burke, L., D. Pyrne, and R. Telford. "Effect of oral creatine supplementation on single-effort sprint performance in elite swimmers." *International Journal of Sport Nutrition* 6 (1996): 222–233.

Casal, D.C. and A.S. Leon. "Failure of caffeine to affect substrate utilization during prolonged running." *Medicine and Science in Sports and Exercise* 17 (1985): 174–179.

Cheng, W., et al. "Beta-hydroxy beta-methylbutyrate increases fatty acid oxidation by muscle cells." *FASEB Journal* 11(3) (1997): A381.

Cole, K., D.L. Costill, R. Starling, et al. "Effect of caffeine ingestion on perception of effort and subsequent work production." *International Journal of Sport Nutrition* 6 (1996): 14–23.

Costill, D.L., G.P. Dalsky, and W.J. Fink. "Effects of caffeine ingestion on metabolism and exercise performance." *Medicine and Science in Sports and Exercise* 10 (1978): 155–158.

DeLanghe, I., et al. "Normal reference values for creatine, creatinine, and carnitine are lower in vegetarians." *Clinical Chemistry* 35 (1989): 26–35.

Dodd, S.L., R.A. Herb, and S.K. Power. "Caffeine and exercise performance." *Sports Medicine* 15 (1993): 14–23.

Essig, D., D.L. Costill, and R.J. Van Handel. "Effects of caffeine ingestion on utilization of muscle glycogen and lipid during leg ergometer cycling." *International Journal of Sports Medicine* 1 (1980): 86–90.

Fahey, T.D. and M.S. Pearl. "The hormonal and perceptive effects of phosphatidylserine administration during two weeks of weight training-induced over-training." *Biological Sport,* in press.

Fisher, S.M., R.G. McMurray, M. Berry, et al. "Influence of caffeine on exercise performance in habitual caffeine users." *International Journal of Sports Medicine* 7 (1986): 276–280.

Gaesser, G.A. and R.G. Rich. "Influence of caffeine on blood lactate response during incremental exercise." *International Journal of Sports Medicine* 6 (1985): 207–211.

Green, A. "Carbohydrate ingestion augments creatine retention during creatine feedings in humans." *Acta Physiologica Scandinavia* 158 (1996): 195–202.

Green, A., et al. "Creatine ingestion augments muscle creatine uptake and glycogen synthesis during carbohydrate feeding in man." *Journal of Physiology* 491 (1996): 63.

Hellsten-Westling, Y., et al. "Decreased resting levels of adenine nucleotides in human skeletal muscle after high-intensity training." *Journal of Applied Physiology* 74(5) (1993): 2523–2528.

Hultman, E.K., et al. "Muscle creatine loading in man." *Journal of Applied Physiology* 81 (1996): 232–237.

Ivy, J. "Effect of pyruvate and dihydroxyacetone on metabolism and aerobic performance." *Medicine and Science in Sports and Exercise* 30 (1998): 837–843.

Ivy, J.L., D.L. Costill, W.J. Fink, et al. "Influence of caffeine and carbohydrate feedings on endurance performance." *Medicine and Science in Sports and Exercise* 11 (1979): 6–11.

Kidd, P.M. *Phosphatidylserine* (New Canaan, CT: Keats Publishing, 1998).

Kreider, R.B. "Creatine supplement: Analysis of ergogenic value, medical safety and concerns." *Journal of Exercise Physiology Online* 1 (1998): 1–11.

Kreider, R., e. al. "Effects of B-HMB supplementation with and without creatine during training on body composition alterations." *FASEB Journal* 11(3) (1997): A374.

Monteleone, P., et al. "Blunting by chronic phosphatidylserine administration of the stress-induced activation of the hypothalamo-pituitary-adrenal axis in healthy men." *European Journal of Clinical Pharmacology* 41 (1992): 385–388.

Monteleone, P., et al. "Effects of phosphatidylserine on the neuroendocrine responses to physical stress in humans." *Neuroendocrinology* 52 (1990): 243–248.

Monteleone, P., et al. "Blunting by chronic phosphatidylserine administration of the stress-induced activation of the hypothalamo-pituitary-adrenal axis." *European Journal of Clinical Pharmacology* 41 (1992): 385–388.

Nissen, S., et al. "Effect of leucine metabolite beta-hydroxy-beta-methylbutyrate on muscle metabolism during resistance training." *Journal of Applied Physiology* 81 (1996): 2095–2104.

Nissen, S., et. al. "Effects of feeding beta-hydroxy beta-methylbutyrate (HMB) on body composition in women." *FASEB Journal* 11(3) (1997): A290.

Passwater, R. *Creatine* (New Canaan, CT: Keats Publishing Inc., 1997), pp. 41–42.

Passwater, R. and J. Fuller. *Building Muscle Mass, Performance and Health with HMB* (New Canaan, CT: Keats Publishing, 1997).

Powers, S., R. Byrd, R. Tulley, et al. "Effects of caffeine ingestion on metabolism and performance during graded exercise." *European Journal of Applied Physiology* 40 (1983): 301–307.

Robertson, R.J., R.T. Stanko, F.L. Goss, et al. "Blood glucose extraction as a mediator of perceived exertion during prolonged exercise." *European Journal of Applied Physiology* 61 (1990): 100–105.

Spriet, L.L. "Caffeine and performance." *International Journal of Sport Nutrition* 5 (1995): S84–S99.

Stanko, R.T., R.J. Robertson, R.J. Spina, et al. "Enhancement of arm exercise endurance capacity with dihydroxyacetone and pyruvate." *Journal of Applied Physiology* 68 (1990): 119–124.

Stanko, R.T., R.J. Robertson, R.W. Galbreath, et al. "Enhanced leg exercise endurance with a high carbohydrate diet and dihydroxyacetone and pyruvate." *Journal of Applied Physiology* 69 (1990): 1651–1656.

Stathis, C., et al. "Influence of sprint training on human skeletal muscle purine nucleotide metabolism." *Journal of Applied Physiology* 76(4) (1994): 1802–1809.

Ternlion, K., et al. "The effect of creatine supplementation on two 700-m maximal running bouts." *International Journal of Sports Nutrition* 7 (1997): 138–143.

Thompson, P.D. and B Franklin. "Creatine supplements face scrutiny: Will users pay later?" *The Physician and Sports Medicine* 26 (1998): 15–23.

Tullson, P. and R. Terjung. "Adenine nucleotide synthesis in exercising and endurance-trained skeletal muscle." *American Journal of Physiology* 261 (1991): C342–C347.

Tullson P., D. Whitlock, and R. Terjung. "Adenine nucleotide degradation in slow-twitch red muscle." *American Journal of Physiology* 258 (1990): C258–C265.

Tullson, P., et al. "IMP metabolism in human skeletal muscle after exhaustive exercise." *Journal of Applied Physiology* 78 (1995) (1): 146–152.

Tullson, P., et al. "IMP reamination to AMP in rat skeletal muscle fiber types." *American Journal of Physiology* 270 (1996): C1067–C1074.

Vanderberghe, K., et al. "Caffeine counteracts the ergogenic action of muscle creatine loading." *Journal of Applied Physiology* 80 (1996): 452–457.

Chapter 14: Nutrition to Delay Fatigue

Anderson, M., et al. "Pre-exercise meal affects ride time to fatigue in trained cyclists." *Journal of the American Dietetic Association* 94 (1994): 1152–1153.

DeMarco, H.M., et al. "Pre-exercise carbohydrate meals application of glycemic index." *Medicine and Science in Sports and Exercise* 31 (1999): 164–170.

Piehl, K. "Time course for refilling of glycogen stores in human muscle fibres following exercise-induced glycogen depletion." *Acta Physiologica Scandinavica* 90 (1974): 297–302.

Pizza, F., et al. "A carbohydrate loading regimen improves high intensity, short duration exercise performance." *International Journal of Sport Science* (1995): 110–116.

Chapter 15: Nonnutritional Approaches to Recovery

Anderson, B. *Stretching* (Bolinas, CA: Shelter Publications, 1980).

Anderson, B., E. Burke, and B. Pearl. *Getting in Shape: Workout Programs for Men & Women* (Bolinas, CA: Shelter Publications, 1994).

Pozeznik, R. *Massage for Cyclists* (Brattleboro, VT: Vitesse Press, 1995).

INDEX

N

Neck stretch, 179

Neutrophils, 83

Newsholme, Eric, 35, 82, 83

Niacin. *See* Vitamin B complex.

Nieman, David, 85, 86

Noakes, Tim, 47

Nonessential amino acids. *See* Amino acids.

Non-heme iron, 138

O

ODIs. *See* Optimum Daily Intakes.

Omega-3 fatty acids. *See* Essential fatty acids.

Omega-6 fatty acids. *See* Essential fatty acids.

Optimum Daily Intakes, 125

Optimum recovery ratio, 67, 72

OR^2. *See* Optimum recovery ratio.

Osteoporosis, 133

OTS. *See* Overtraining syndrome.

Overheating, 27–30

Overtraining
    dangers of, 47–49
    preventing complications of, 49
    symptoms of, 48

Overtraining syndrome, 47, 82

Oxidants. *See* Free radicals.

Oxidative stress. *See* Free-radical damage.

P

Pantothenic acid. *See* Vitamin B complex.

PDIs. *See* Performance Daily Intakes.

Performance Daily Intakes, 124, 126

Phosphatidylserine, supplementing with, 150–151

Phospholipids, 76

Phosphorus, 134–135

Physical training, protein intake and, 91–92

Polysaccharides, 109

Polyunsaturated fatty acids, 112

Potassium, 55, 57–58, 62, 135, 136

Protein, 17–18, 89, 98, 107, 115
    as a fuel source, 90–93
    dietary guidelines for, 116–117
    enhancing synthesis of, 93–95
    incomplete, 115
    insulin and, 67–68, 93
    requirements for athletes, 91–93
    supplemental forms of, 117–121

Prothrombin, 129

Pruitt, Andy, 169

Avery Publishing Group
120 Old Broadway
Garden City Park, NY 11040

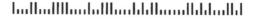

Avery Publishing Group
120 Old Broadway
Garden City Park, NY 11040